WIDE AWAKE, CLEAR HEADED, AND REFRESHED . . .

MEDICAL HYPNOANALYSIS IN ACTION

3-11-99
Samuel,
Thanks a lot!
Regan Elliott

WIDE AWAKE, CLEAR HEADED, AND REFRESHED . . .

Medical Hypnoanalysis in Action

Hypnoanalysis: A tested and proven system for strengthening skills, boosting performance, learning to love, and improving all dimensions of your life.

Ryan Elliott, M.S.W.

Relaxed Books
Winfield, Illinois
1991

Project Editors: Gene Owens and Tom Watson
Text Design and Compositor: Ginger M. Schultz, G. Schultz Publications Production
Cover Design: Lori A. Evans
Copy Editor/Proofreader: Patricia K. Kummer

First Edition

Library of Congress Catalog Card Number: 91-090503
Elliott, Ryan
Wide Awake, Clear Headed, and Refreshed . . .
1. Hypnosis—Psychology 2. Hypnoanalysis
ISBN 0-9615140-0-0 soft cover
September 1991

Workshops and Lectures

Ryan Elliott offers seminars, lectures, and training workshops on topics related to hypnosis and hypnoanalysis. He also conducts groups on interpersonal skills, intimacy, and conflict resolution. If you would like to attend one of Ryan Elliott's upcoming lectures or workshops or invite him to speak in your area, please write to Relaxed Books.

Attention:
Educational Institutions, Libraries, Hospitals, and Retail Outlets

Relaxed Books publications are available at quantity discounts with bulk purchase for educational or sales promotional use. For information, please write to the address below.

You can order any Relaxed Books publication. Simply send title and retail price, plus $3.00 per order to cover mailing and handling for each book desired.
Enclose check, money order, or VISA/MasterCard number and send to:

Thunderbird Circle Publications
Relaxed Books Division
P.O. Box 535
Winfield, IL 60190 **Or call 1-800-421-2717.**

This book is dedicated

to my daughter Julie

and my grandson Travis.

Acknowledgements and Author's Notes

I wish to thank the following people for their help and loving support: Tom Watson, who unfortunately died during the editing process; The American Academy of Medical Hypnoanalysts and especially Patricia Honiotes, M.S.; Dr. George Honiotes, M.D.; Alan Matez, D.O.; John Scott, Sr., Ph.D.; Earl Taylor, Th.D.; Mary Kullman-Taylor, M.S.; Dr. Dan Zelling, M.D.; the late Dr. William Jennings Bryan, Jr., M.D.—a man I would have been honored to have known; Nido Quebein and Gene Owens; my friends Larry Todryk, Renée Ryan, Wendy Wein, Caren Musaraca, Mary Jo Curran, Lori Kuwik; my employees Rae Nitz, Elva Belles, Ami Burgess, Kim Kosatka; Lori Evans for her illustrations and cover design; and the others who have helped but whose names escape me now.

Most of all, I thank my clients who have volunteered their stories, backgrounds, and intimate details of their lives to make this book a reality. In keeping clients' identities disguised due to the confidential nature of the material, names have been changed and other telltale facts distorted for protection without diluting the basic elements of the cases. In several situations, the third person personal pronoun *he* is used and should be read as *he or she*.

My intention was to present an overall description of the hypnoanalytic process as well as present other useful information on subconscious management. For brevity, some of the concepts are underdeveloped. Some of the difficult ideas have been simplified for expediency. A curious reader can research the bibliographic sources cited in the chapter notes. However, what I know at this point is that *Wide Awake, Clear Headed, and Refreshed . . .* is the only book written on medical hypnoanalysis. The spiritual aspect of the treatment was especially shortchanged. Since this part of medical hypnoanalysis plays such a large and absolutely necessary role in the treatment, I apologize and hope you will look for my next book, which will include thorough coverage of this topic.

I have made every effort to document my sources. Full information from some citations, however, is missing. Also, some quotations—especially treasured by me are not cited in the chapter notes. I have gleaned them over the years from books, articles, speeches, and seminars.

CONTENTS

INTRODUCTION

ARE YOU IN CONTROL?

Let us define mental health
as the adjustment
of human beings
to the world
and to each other
with a maximum of
effectiveness and happiness.
Not just efficiency
or just contentment —
or the grace
of obeying
the rules of the game
cheerfully.
It is all these together.
It is the ability
to maintain an even temper,
an alert intelligence,
socially considerate behavior,
and a happy disposition.
This, I think, is a healthy mind.

—Dr. Karl A. Menninger

ARE YOU IN CONTROL?

Life is a do-it-yourself project. Our thoughts and feelings are the tools through which we construct our life-project. Our circumstances are the products of our thoughts and feelings. Especially those thoughts and feelings forgotten and lodged in our subconscious mind. We have to be careful what we think because we can set ourselves up for what we get. We do, in fact, create reality through our thinking. In other words, we get what we expect to get, especially when our expectations stem from fear. Fear calls into existence that which we're afraid of.

The subconscious mind is the mechanism behind everyday existence. Think about it: Everything you believe and emotionally embrace—whether positive or negative—has manifested itself in your life—everything! We create our realities based on how we think and program our minds. The philosophy of personal responsibility means that our subconscious, fear-based programming influences the events in our lives here and now. By personal responsibility, we mean that others—our parents, our society, our friends and lovers—are not responsible for our circumstances. Personal responsibility means that the buck stops with us. Our subconscious minds have accepted suggestions and dictated our feelings and behaviors—those wanted as well as those unwanted. By discovering our programming from earlier periods of life, by bringing it into our awareness, by understanding and reinterpreting it, then letting go of it, we can free ourselves to be the way we really want to be. We can take charge of our do-it-yourself lives.

You develop personal power by balancing and directing your creative energy. You can make your life different if you want to because you have the power to bring about change in yourself and in your environment. You've created what you have now, and you can make your life come out any way you want. *Wide Awake, Clear Headed, and Refreshed* . . . will help you discover why you are where you are and how to get where you want to be. Through medical hypnoanalysis and by developing your mind power, you can change.

This book is for you if:

- You have a habit or behavior that is getting the best of you.
- Your self-esteem isn't what it should be.
- You have good habits you would like to strengthen.

- You're depressed, anxious, or fearful.
- You want to become more competent, confident, and successful in your chosen endeavors.
- You experience useless guilt.
- You want to be more at ease in situations that currently make you uncomfortable.
- You want to know how to connect to God or your higher power.
- You want to unlock mental powers that you have never used.
- You've had difficulty knowing who you are.
- You want to know more about the role your past has played in your present existence.

Hypnoanalysis is analysis of subconscious programming through the use of hypnosis; hypnosis is a natural state of mind. Hypnosis opens the door to the subconscious; analysis opens a person's understanding to the cause of the problem, and the analyst redirects the energy toward a solution—hence, the term, hypnoanalysis.

Although I will discuss the history of hypnosis and hypnoanalysis in Chapter Two, let me just say here that hypnosis was recognized by the American Medical Association in 1958 as a legitimate approach to solving medical problems. More and more doctors and their patients recognize the idea that the mind and body interact to cause illness and behavioral problems. Mind and body are integrated parts of a whole; a change in one part affects the other—the chicken-or-egg dilemma.

Hypnoanalysis is a comfortable, reassuring way to help you change your mind about yourself, about the people you relate to, and about the world. We really are evolution in process. Through hypnosis, we concentrate our minds and affect our realities. By affecting our minds and by changing ourselves, we can change our evolution.

Hypnosis is one of the best tools through which you can accomplish understanding and change—a pen with which you can write a new life plan. By harnessing your mind power through hypnosis, you can raise yourself out of poverty, unhappiness, misery, alcoholism, sexual problems, and drug addiction. You can give up smoking, lose weight, and overcome fears and phobias.

Medical hypnoanalysis solves emotional and psychological problems by going after the underlying causes. The difficult part of the process is the analysis of the subconscious, reaching into the subconscious mind and pulling out negative suggestions that have lodged there, nullifying them and replacing them with positive suggestions. That's where a qualified professional hypnoanalyst can help. And although hypnoanalysis is not magical or a panacea, it's a powerful method for improving the human condition.

Remember that the subconscious automatically remembers events from early periods of our lives—memories that affect who we are and what we do today. We may need the help of a professional hypnoanalyst to recall and review memories. It's important to remember that subconscious memories are not readily available to waking consciousness. The hypnotic state creates an inroad to the subconscious.

Recognizing the underlying cause of an attitude or feeling may be all that is needed to erase its power over us. However, the simple understanding of why we eat too much, why we smoke, why we are afraid of heights, or whatever, may not be adequate to eliminate some problem feelings or problem behaviors. In such cases, hypnoanalysis can be helpful. While we are in a hypnotic state, we are more receptive to a therapist's positive suggestions to reprogram our thinking and change those problem behaviors.

Therapy is a phenomenon, not a fact. It's like the difference between a hero and heroism. We can watch a person being or acting the hero. But even though we know that heroism exists, we cannot see it. Like therapy, heroism is a phenomenon. Something happens between client and therapist that cannot be quantified or measured, but its results can be felt and observed. The word "therapy" comes from the Greek word *therapeia*, which means, literally, "the work of the gods."

In hypnoanalysis, a trained therapist uses gentle suggestion to help remove limiting beliefs and construct positive, life-affirming ones. Whatever goal is set through therapy is decided upon and self-directed by the client with the therapist acting as a guide. Through the following steps, a hypnoanalyst guides you in uncovering the origin of your problem, undoing the subconscious knot, and freeing yourself to live a healthier, more productive life:

1. Relaxation. By learning to relax and let the mind go, you can concentrate and allow an opening to your subconscious. Then, the next step becomes possible.

2. Realization. Difficulties stem from negative thinking and feeling—suggestions. By realizing the source and power of your programming, you can learn to restructure those problem attitudes and create the outlook you desire.

3. Reeducation. Reeducation helps you recognize the difference between the underlying cause from the past and the conscious problem-belief. When the underlying cause is part of your past, it can be removed by direct suggestion and by realizing the past is past and recognizing that the need for the problem has passed too.

4. Rehabilitation. Through hypnotherapy, you will get new information and positive suggestions, and will have time to correct bad habits—time to rehabilitate your thinking and practice your new thought patterns.

5. Reassurance. You gain reassurance through a number of avenues. Family or friends may indicate that you're getting better. You experience a decrease in symptoms. Your analyst will take advantage of any change, no matter how slight, to remind you of the improvement.

6. Repetition. Repetition is necessary to implant positive suggestions in the soil of your subconscious. The more you repeat something, the more permanently implanted it becomes in your mind.

7. Reinforcement. By developing your skill in self-hypnosis, you will be able to support the positive suggestions you've received from the analyst, enabling you to continue the growth begun in the office.

8. Responsibility. Once the first seven steps have been accomplished, accepting responsibility for your life is the natural outcome.

This approach to problem solving owes a debt to Freud, Mesmer, and Dr. William Jennings Bryan, Jr., M.D. Yet, researchers have for several years been validating the concepts through their clinical observations.

From an informational reading exercise, you can turn this book into a transformational experience. It will:

- Acquaint you with the process of hypnoanalysis.
- Instruct you in inducing a self-hypnotic state.
- Show you how to program your mind for improved, increased performance.
- Challenge you to take control of your circumstances and in as little as 30 days create change.

Wide Awake, Clear Headed, and Refreshed . . . will show you how to make things happen to you instead of just watching them happen to others. While deep-seated problems will require aid from a qualified hypnoanalyst, you can effect many changes in your life through the practice of self-suggestion in hypnosis. As you learn more about the power of your subconscious mind, you can see and feel how suggestion and self-hypnosis can improve the quality of your life, both physically and emotionally.

It's up to you, just as your entire life is up to you. Remember, you are in control. Or are you? If not, it's high time to take control.

CHAPTER ONE

A CHANCE TO UNDERSTAND YOUR TRANCE

The
purpose
of life
after all,
is to live it,
to taste the experience
to the utmost, to reach out
eagerly and without fear for
newer and richer experiences.

—Eleanor Roosevelt

YOUR LIFE IS UNIQUE

Have you ever thought about what makes you "you"? You came into this world without any idea of yourself at all, in neutral. Your conscious mind was a blank slate. Genetics aside, you were no different from any other newborn infant in your ability to perceive and respond to your reality. You were born with two fears, the fears of falling and loud noises, plus all of your physical needs.

Instantly, that began to change. From the first moment of your life, you started on a unique, individual journey. Your mind started recognizing and retaining memories of your varied experiences. From infancy through the present, the tracings on your mind's "slate" have filled one day after another.

By now, you've accumulated literally thousands of yesterdays and a wealth of knowledge to apply to the rest of your future. Those experiences are what make you a unique person. While people in a given peer group might share similar experiences, no two people in the world have perceived identical pasts. Because of that, even individuals sharing the same developmental experience might walk away with different perceptions. Three witnesses of an automobile accident, for example, might sound as if they were describing three totally different events. The reality of the accident does not change, but that reality is perceived differently by each of the three witnesses.

The old story of five blind men describing an elephant also comes to mind. The first one held the elephant's trunk and declared the animal to resemble a hose. The second held its tail and insisted that an elephant was really like a rope. The third touched the leg and concluded that the animal was like a tree. The fourth touched an ear and believed that the creature amazingly resembled a huge leaf. The fifth, touching the massive side, concluded that his companions were all wrong: An elephant, obviously, was like a wall. None of them changed the reality that stood before them. But each perceived the reality from a different perspective.

THE WORKINGS OF THE SUBCONSCIOUS MIND

Since you are the product of your experiences, your past plays a strong part in determining how you perceive every incident in your life. Your subconscious mind is the storehouse of all your experiences. It records every hurt and trauma you experience, even while the conscious mind chooses to forget life's earlier incidents. It is a warehouse of memories and lessons that you can apply to the present and future. Yet, even more important to the quality of your future than the memories you've accumulated is the power of the subconscious mind in which they're stored.

Although the subconscious is subservient to the conscious mind, it is much more than a storage container for memories. The subconscious controls the nervous system, which controls the operation of the body's involuntary functions. Often called the irrational or reactive mind, it actually keeps you alive. Without your subconscious, your heart, lungs, kidneys, and other vital organs would not function. The subconscious can make the body move into many unhealthy coping actions.

Frank, a 50-year-old, two-pack-a-day smoker, started puffing as a teenager because it was the "cool" thing to do at the time. Now, of course, he's hooked. His nicotine addiction is a physical reality, but there's something else that makes cigarettes so hard to give up. Every time he lights up, Frank's subconscious still tells him he looks like James Dean, that cool, idealized image he tried to live up to as a teenager. The old memory sent to the subconscious keeps coming back to keep him lighting up one cigarette after another.

The subconscious also is responsible for a lot of other functions. We experience life through our five senses. We see, hear, taste, touch, and smell. We may or may not enjoy our experiences, based on our perceptions, which trigger our emotions, located in our subconscious minds.

The subconscious, including superconsciousness, is sometimes referred to as the right brain, although it is not conclusively located in the right hemisphere of the brain. It is responsible for creativity. All literary and musical compositions, creative inventions, and original ideas are the products of the creative, subconscious mind. The same is true for intuition. When an incident occurs that you sensed beforehand, your extrasensory perception (ESP)—that is to say your right-brain subconscious—has been at work.

Does this mean that the subconscious has magical powers? Yes and no, depending upon how you define "magical." The subconscious does have a lot of power—more power than most people even dream they have at their disposal.

Creativity, intuition, and imagination are functions of the subconscious mind, and the results in reality depend upon the information stored in the subconscious. When your intuition leads you to predict someone's next move, it's because your subconscious mind is reviewing its knowledge of that individual and responding with a logical or expected reaction. When you imagine a particular scenario, you are creating a thought based on your knowledge of similar settings. For example, even if you've never been to the Adirondack Mountains, you still could develop a mental picture of what you think they look like, based on your experience with other mountains. Whether your mental image really looks like the Adirondacks is not important here. Right or wrong, your imagination—in your subconscious—still creates a visual image.

With 90 percent of your brain devoted to the subconscious mind, you can imagine how much information you can store in it. Some experts believe that the average human being has enough brain power to master some 40 foreign languages, commit a complete set of encyclopedias to memory, and even complete full-course requirements from a dozen universities. This is because the average brain, which weighs just under four pounds, is able to house up to two quintillion bits of information. In a figure, that is 2,000,000,000,000,000,000. McDonald's at its current rate won't sell that many hamburgers for another 875 million years—give or take a few centuries, of course.

THE WORKINGS OF THE CONSCIOUS MIND

Before anything can be stored in your subconscious mind, it must first pass the objective or conscious mind. The conscious mind, which deals with outward things, is logical, mathematical, and orderly. Because the conscious mind feeds information to the subconscious, everything you've ever learned or experienced is stored in your subconscious mind. Since 90 percent of the brain is devoted to the subconscious mind, this means that only 10 percent is involved with conscious thought.

One can't help developing an appreciation for the power of the subconscious. The conscious mind is analytical by nature and controls conscious activities such as thinking, speaking, writing, arithmetic, planning, organizing, judgment, and reading. The conscious mind, through imagination, is often called the gateway to the subconscious because only the conscious mind can access information stored in the subconscious and bridge the gap between reality and the subconscious mind. You are using your conscious mind right now to read the words on this page. When you recall this information tomorrow, it will be because your conscious mind has retrieved it from your subconscious storage department.

Because the conscious mind can retrieve information from the subconscious, we can function as productive human beings. Even though reading requires conscious activity, the knowledge of vowel sounds, phonetics, and word definitions stored in your subconscious allows you to read quickly, without conscious thought. The same applies to mathematics. It requires conscious ability, for instance, to multiply 365 by 4. If you've committed multiplication tables to memory—your subconscious—you know that 5 times 4 equals 20, 6 times 4 equals 24, and 3 times 4 equals 12. After adding and carrying the appropriate figures, your conscious mind can determine the answer: 1,460.

Almost everything we do involves cooperation between our conscious and subconscious minds. Although the subconscious is receptive to suggestion, nothing goes into the subconscious against the will or evaluation of the conscious mind. Your subconscious cannot make comparisons or judgments. It does not reason through information or determine truth, but simply reacts to impressions transmitted to it from the conscious mind.

The formula or instructions for any action you execute repeatedly become fixed in your subconscious, and the information becomes available upon conscious command. Routine actions from tying your shoelaces to operating a motor vehicle become second nature through the power of the subconscious. So does operating a typewriter, computer, calculator, or any other machine you regularly use. The advertising industry implants its messages in the public's subconscious mind through repetition. This is why you can remember popular commercials years after the media have stopped running them. If you can recall things you learned in grade school—or even yesterday—it is because the conscious mind has retrieved it from the subconscious.

PUSH THE RIGHT BUTTON AND OUT COMES THE INFORMATION

Why do you sometimes have trouble recalling something? For example, you might have a clear picture in your conscious mind of the face of a former schoolteacher, even though you can't recall his or her name. Or sometimes you can remember the first two lines of a poem or a song, but you can't remember the rest. Does that mean that the information is gone? No. Considering the almost limitless storage capacity of your subconscious mind, it's highly unlikely it will ever be filled to capacity.

Much of the information about our past is not readily available, however, because the conscious mind does not have the proper stimulus to retrieve it. For example, the poem you cannot remember might come back to you if someone gave you the first word or two of the forgotten portion. Or the name of the instructor might come to you instantly if someone gave you the initials. No information in your subconscious is ever "forgotten." Obscure information deep in the subconscious often needs a "hint," a priming, to bring it back into the conscious mind.

In contrast, there are experiences you can easily remember. Both happy and sad memories of close relationships never seem to fade. The same is true for memories of very pleasant or very miserable events. That is because information of high emotional impact is instantly and firmly committed to your subconscious mind.

PERCEIVED TRUTHS TRANSLATE INTO BELIEFS

The adult who craves sweets may be allergic or may have acquired the craving as a child. Without self-discipline, such a craving can lead to an overweight problem by the time the child reaches adulthood.

Recognizing the disadvantages of obesity, a person might consciously decide that sugar is not a good thing at all and that it should be avoided whenever possible. By this time, though, the subconscious may be hooked. Cutting out sweets isn't an easy thing to do.

This is similar to what may happen when a person starts smoking, except that nearly all smokers will tell you that cigarettes taste terrible at first. Still, new smokers consciously light up (for reasons that we'll discuss in detail in Chapter Seven). In time, the cigarettes begin to taste good until, one day, they are too good to give up. The subconscious is hooked.

I've dealt with many clients who have wanted to give up sweets or cigarettes. They have sought my services after finding they couldn't win the battle without professional help. Although they had consciously decided they wanted to kick their psychological—if not physical—addictions, they found that their subconscious minds put up too tough a battle. Once your subconscious mind establishes a bit of information as a "truth"—that sugar or cigarettes are good, for example—there is often hell to pay if you try to change that position. That is why ex-smokers often refer to their first days (if not weeks) without cigarettes as going "cold turkey." The psychological torture that the subconscious inflicts can be too much for the conscious mind to bear. Many would-be sugar or nicotine quitters finally cave in and indulge themselves with a vengeance. They consciously realize the undesirable consequences of resuming their habits. Yet, that realization makes no difference to the subconscious. Only a dose of what it is accustomed to receiving can satisfy it. When the conscious and the subconscious minds are in conflict, the conscious mind will almost always lose the battle. Susan's[1] story illustrates the personal trauma she experienced in her attempt to lose weight.

Sweets Were Her Fix

"'Dear God . . . PLEASE make this the last time,' I thought, as I drove to the local bakery.

"I was already stuffed from a full lunch at a nearby restaurant. But being stuffed was irrelevant. I wanted more. I knew a few sweet rolls would go down real well and I'd still be on time for my 3 P.M. appointment with Ryan Elliott.

"I was desperately hoping the yo-yo cycles would end, but I was VERY skeptical. How could he do what I had been unable to do since the age of 7?

"But I had made up my mind that this was to be the last binge. I bought two doughnuts, two creme horns and one petit-four pastry and zoomed back to the car. I headed toward Winfield, shoving the 'illegal' goodies into my mouth, watching crumbs flying everywhere as I ate.

"What an awful trip. Sweets were my fix. For me the 'drug of choice' was Hostess Suzy-Qs and anything from the bakery. Compulsive eating—or compulsive bingeing—had become a way of life.

"I wanted OUT.

"Why couldn't I be normal, eat normally and control my weight like the rest of the world? I was plenty miserable by the time I pulled into the parking lot and entered the office.

"I'd tried therapy before. 'What would make this time different?' I wondered, as I was escorted to a small consultation room.

"His secretary took some pretty mundane information, which she wrote on my file folder, and told me to wait for Ryan.

"Several minutes elapsed and I really wondered, 'What am I doing here?' I had a real uneasy feeling. 'Maybe I'm coming down from my sugar high. I'm an invincible person. I can stand anything . . . even this.' I was already frightened at the thought of admitting I was out of control and this 'superwoman' couldn't solve her own eating problem.

"Ryan began to take my case history, probing all sorts of areas that I, quite frankly, would rather not talk about. He asked about my childhood, my parents (both deceased), siblings (none), and my sex life.

"What sex life? People who are fat and ugly don't have sex lives. He should know better.

"Finally, he explained that the program would take 30 sessions, twice a week for 15 weeks. He strongly recommended an up-front payment so when the 'going got rough' I'd have a financial investment and would continue the program. I made a mental note that I'd have absolutely no problem. I'm strong. I'm invincible. He wouldn't get to me—others, yes—me, no.

"The first hypnosis treatment followed.

"Blindfolded, headset in place, vibrating chair turned on. I was ready. That first session was an introduction to hypnosis and how to do self-hypnosis to support the office treatments.

"I made two appointments for the coming week before leaving.

"I wanted to succeed more than anything. And, I was MOTIVATED. I stayed on a very reasonable eating plan and dropped two pounds by my next visit.

"Then came the visit that was to change my life.

"It was Friday. Time for the word-association test. I was hypnotized as usual. By now, the blindfold, headset, and vibrating easy chair were becoming routine. Then, oh! Oh! The chair stopped its normal vibrating and there was an awful silence. And, I heard Ryan's voice.

"Simultaneously, my stomach tightened and I had a sickening feeling. 'Oh, no! This guy is going to get to know the real me.'

"I can't describe how terrifying the thought of full self-disclosure was. Ryan gave me a word and I was to respond with the first word or thought that came to mind. And, oh, the words! I was mortified at my responses.

"I left the office thinking, 'I NEVER want to come back.'

"'Awkward,' 'embarrassed,' 'horrified' only hint at the way I felt. My depression grew with every passing hour. I drove home. Had dinner. Went to bed. I was even more depressed when I awoke. I struggled to get out of bed. 'If I go to my exercise class, I'll feel better,' I thought. My body was sluggish. I didn't want to exercise. I didn't want to eat. I didn't want to do ANYTHING. The feeling in my gut was awful—a feeling I'd never experienced before.

"This had to be a severe case of depression: I certainly had all the symptoms. I sat on the stairs by the phone and stared into space for an hour.

"Two voices were fighting in my head: Superwoman kept saying, 'This is ridiculous. You can control any situation. Get hold of yourself.'

"The other voice said, 'You feel awful. You need reassurance. Call Ryan.'

"I picked up the phone. And put it back. The pattern repeated for several minutes.

"Finally, I realized that I was not Superwoman, that I very, very much needed someone, and that someone was Ryan. He was the only person who would know what was going on in my head and heart.

"Finally, I made probably the most significant phone call of my life. Being Superwoman is an awesome responsibility to carry all the time. It was wonderful to have someone be there and take the burden.

"Ryan assured me I wasn't crazy and the depression would go away. He asked what I was feeling. I'd just begun to learn what it was to FEEL anything.

"At that moment, I realized that I ate to hide from the world and from my own feelings. Food was my only friend. I used food to escape from life and to keep people and experiences out.

"When the overeating was removed from my life, I began to experience emotions and feelings—like other people experience every day.

"Suddenly, it occurred to me that if I could feel depression, I could also feel joy—a delightful thought to consider.

"Ryan got through the wall of fat and emotion. At times the process was painful, but it was a necessary part of making me well. Although the therapy was not always pleasant, the benefits were a thousandfold better than the pain, so I continued with the treatment, gaining insights into my reasons for eating. Negative suggestions which contributed to my desire to overeat were removed through hypnosis. I ate reasonable-to-small quantities of food, and, surprise, I was FULL!!!

"Through hypnosis, Ryan also worked on improving my self-esteem and confidence. Very slowly I began to emerge from behind the wall of fat. My outlook shifted to POSITIVE. I started loving myself. I learned to give and receive emotional feelings.

"Does the story have a happy ending? Well, this is real life, but I think so. Working with Ryan, I lost 27 pounds, making me a total of 50 pounds thinner than last year. I feel wonderful. Compliments abound.

"The best part of the change, though, is what I gained: self-love and self-esteem. I'm not perfect, but I don't expect to be. I just have to be me, and now, I know that's ok.

"I certainly don't need food in the addictive way I did before. Therapy is a slow process—a little bit of insight at a time. The benefits have been overwhelmingly positive in my life. It's fun to get high on people and friends rather than on food.

"The world looks different and wonderful because Ryan and I changed ME! God heard my prayer. Thank you, God."

Susan

If You Think It's True

Much like Susan, many people go through life acting on "beliefs" that aren't true. Reality isn't as important as *perceived* reality. Individual reality is an extension or projection of consciousness. Many people in the world today do not live up to their potential because they believe they lack certain abilities. They believe they aren't intelligent, capable, skilled, or talented enough to achieve their ambitions. Individuals who believe they are inadequate usually are. A conscious belief eventually becomes committed to a person's subconscious mind—regardless of whether the belief reflects true or false information.

Once you develop an individual belief, you generally react or adapt to it. People who suffer from anorexia nervosa commit a slow form of suicide. They literally starve themselves to death because they believe they are too fat. Among tribes and cults that practice voodoo, there are documented cases of people who died within a half hour after a witch doctor placed a spell or curse upon them. There was no foul play involved. The individuals simply believed they were going to die while under the spell of the curse, and they did. These people programmed their minds to engineer their own deaths.

So doesn't it stand to reason that if the mind can be programmed to engineer death, it can also be programmed to enhance life? Most emphatically, it can! The subconscious mind is strictly impartial. It doesn't care whether you live or die, succeed or fail. It will simply function the way you program it to function.

The choice is yours, and if you've chosen to improve the quality of your life, then keep reading. Otherwise, stop now and don't waste your time. I will show you how it is done through suggestion, self-hypnosis, and the hypnoanalytic process.

THE HIERARCHY OF HUMAN NEEDS

First, let's talk about what motivates human beings. Psychologist Abraham Maslow identified five levels of motivation, which he called the "hierarchy of human needs." According to Maslow, every person starts at the bottom of this hierarchy and works upward through the levels as they progress through life. Only after mastering the lowest level will they focus on another, he contends, and, if at any time security on a lower level is threatened, the individual will drop back and reestablish there before moving up the ladder.

Let's take a look at these five levels.

1. Survival. When our physical survival is in question, nothing else matters. People will work long and hard to obtain food, water, clothing, and shelter. These are the basics of life, and it's hard to become excited about lofty ambitions or social standing when you're hungry and need to work to earn money for your next meal.

2. Security. Once survival is assured, people usually concentrate on their security—survival on a long-term basis. Security translates into peace of mind, safety, stability, savings, a nest egg so that survival is not threatened. It is difficult to find peace if you are constantly concerned with whether you and your family will eat regularly.

3. Social. Only after assuring their survival and establishing security do people turn toward developing relationships for social gratification, for love, and for a sense of belonging. Most people develop "support systems" for emotional needs ranging from spiritual growth to recreational activities.

4. Ego. Once people satisfy their basic physical and social needs, Maslow says, they are ready to turn their attention to gratifying their egos, gaining recognition. They direct their efforts toward becoming good at what they do so others will notice and approve. People work to satisfy ego needs on the job, in their relationships, and in community and volunteer arenas.

5. Self-actualization. After meeting all other needs, people then are free to turn their attention toward self-fulfillment, satisfying their greatest ambitions, doing not just what it takes to survive or even to have a good life, but what they really want to do. Not everyone in life reaches a level at which he or she can do the things that give him or her most pleasure.

Generally, a person's rise through these levels will not be steady but will involve stops and starts—a couple of steps forward, and one or more backward. Also, there is no guarantee that once an individual achieves a certain level, he or she can forget about that one and focus on challenges further up the developmental ladder. Jerky progress is the norm. For example, a person working toward self-actualization might fall all the way back to working toward survival should he or she get wiped out in a stock market crash or a bad investment.

It doesn't matter so much what levels you have reached in the hierarchy. More important is that you be continually challenged and involved and keep moving toward self-actualization. Your motivation will be controlled by the difference between where you feel you are in your climb and where you would eventually like to be.

THE ORDER OF IMPORTANCE

The late Dr. William Jennings Bryan, Jr., M.D., cofounder of the American Institute of Hypnosis, also developed a hierarchical scale. Bryan's assessment of what is important to human beings varied greatly from Maslow's, however.

Bryan, a medical doctor, psychologist, lawyer, and hypnoanalyst, stressed the following forms of survival and their relative importance to human beings:

1. Spiritual survival. An individual's connection to God, to an infinite power, or to a universal intelligence topped Bryan's list of important factors. While admitting that earthly physical well-being is important, Bryan insists that physical security pales in comparison to spiritual well-being. He contrasted Maslow's basic survival level of security to spiritual well-being through Jesus Christ's words, "What good will it be for a man if he gains the whole world, yet forfeits his soul?"[2] Even if you don't believe that your spirit will survive for all eternity, there is still value in respecting and practicing truth, he contended. People will give their lives for someone or something they love, whether it is a person, a country, or a belief. The most miserable people in any society, Bryan said, are those who live lives based on physical survival only.

2. Analytical or mind survival. Next in importance is our ability to make our way in the world, develop self-esteem and establish personal identity. The ability to reason, to discern, and to exercise judgment is of utmost importance, second only to our spiritual survival. As I mentioned earlier, the left brain, or conscious mind, is analytical by nature. It controls such activities as thinking, speaking, writing, arithmetic, planning, organizing, judgment, and reading. A fear much worse than death for many people is the loss of analytical powers, which would turn them into "vegetables."

3. Physical survival. With our mental and emotional faculties assured, physical survival is next on the list of priorities. A major fear with people as they age is that they will lose their physical abilities while their minds are still alert. Physical survival was Maslow's number one priority, you will recall. The fact that smoking is a threat to physical survival does not prevent great numbers of people from puffing away. Using Bryan's order of importance, the personal enjoyment or emotional satisfaction gained from smoking would not outweigh the activity's potential physical harm. Physical survival has three components: air, water, and food. A person can go without air for only moments, water for a few days, and food for a month or so.

4. Territorial survival. As we go through life, we stake out certain "territories" that become very much a part of our identities. Our homes, our jobs, and our social outlets are territories that we won't give up without a fight—unless we have already secured new territories to replace them. This motivational level corresponds to Maslow's security and social levels.

5. Sexual survival. Surprisingly, sexual survival is lowest in importance to most people. Despite America's apparent obsession with sexual activity, as manifested by the mass media, it ranks on the bottom of the list. Although we might not like the idea of survival without sex, most people would agree that they would give up sex before giving up their identities, their bodies, their minds, or their spirits. Given the choice between a meal or sex, a hungry person will opt for the meal.

Now, with some idea of what motivates you and of what you hold important, let me ask you a question: Could your life be better than it is now? You are the only person who can change it. External events that affect your life often are beyond your control. However, the quality of your life is of your own making. Your personality, your health, your marital and employment status, and your social standing are all within your control.

With hypnosis and the God-given power of your mind, you can change undesired behaviors, feelings, thoughts, whatever. Whether it is getting up early in the morning or developing greater creativity, learning to love yourself more or changing addictive behavior, hypnosis and self-suggestion can help you change your way of life for the better.

First, however, it's important that you know more about what hypnoanalysis is and about the exciting personality changes that people can make once they are aware of the true cause of their problems. Recognizing and releasing negative suggestions and repressed emotions will result in great changes in your life. Chapter Two explains more about this science and its practice.

Key Concepts

- Genetics aside, at birth you were similar to any other newborn in your ability to perceive and respond to reality and in your capability to develop your God-given ability to choose.
- Since you are the product of your experiences, your past plays a strong part in determining how you perceive each incident in your life.
- Your subconscious mind has stored all your experiences. It records every hurt and trauma a person experiences, even if the conscious brain chooses to forget life's uglier incidents.
- The subconscious, which includes the superconscious, is responsible for creativity.
- Creativity, intuition, and imagination are functions of the subconscious mind, and the results of these functions depend upon the information stored in the subconscious.
- The conscious mind is analytical by nature and controls conscious activities, such as thinking, speaking, writing, arithmetic, planning, organizing, judgment, and reading.
- When the conscious and the subconscious minds are in conflict, the subconscious mind will almost always win out.
- Reality is not as important as *perceived* reality.
- The subconscious mind is strictly impartial. It doesn't care whether you succeed or fail. It will simply function the way it has been programmed, or the way you program it now.
- Through hypnosis and natural mind power, you can change undesired behaviors, feelings, and thoughts and adopt new ones.
- We live according to our survival in the following areas of life, in descending order of importance:
  1. Spiritual (love)
  2. Identity (self-esteem)
  3. Physical
  4. Territorial (property, money, etc.)
  5. Sexual

Growth Exercise

1. Cite examples of how your past experiences that you know about are influencing your life now. ______________________________
____
____
2. Remember a time when your subconscious mind solved a problem with a spontaneous creative solution? ______________________________
____
3. Did you ever have an ESP experience? ______________________________
4. Name a feeling, behavior, or pattern you have that goes against rational thought? ______________________________
5. What or whom would you give your life for? ______________________________
____

NOTE: Use your answers for more understanding of your subconscious at work.

CHAPTER TWO

THE TRUTH IS SAFER THAN FICTION

To look is one thing;
To see what you look at
is another.
To understand what you see
is a third.
To learn
from what you understand
is still something else.
But to act on what you learn
is all that really matters.

—*Anonymous*

COUNT DRACULA: THE BLACK-CAPED HYPNOTIST

Hollywood melodramas have injured the reputation of hypnosis the same as yellow journalism did to the reputation of newspapers. The corrupt, unscrupulous hypnotist[1] has been the stock villain of many a melodrama. The plots are more or less the same.

The scheming hypnotist enlists the aid of an unwitting subject to do his evil bidding. Most often, murder is the crime. The unwitting subject is hypnotized without his consent or even his knowledge. Then the hypnotist hands him a knife and tells him whom to stab. The subject carries out the deadly instructions. With the victim dead, the hypnotist brings the subject back to reality. The subject emerges with no memory of having committed murder, thus making him the perfect stooge the next time the hypnotist wants someone killed.

Thank goodness this is fiction—and outrageous fiction at that. Because of these melodramas and flamboyant stage shows, which should be billed as "hype-nosis," several classic hypnosis myths persist.

BACK TO REALITY

Let's set the record straight. First, hypnosis is not a sleepwalking state. A hypnotized person is aware of everything that is happening. In fact, hypnosis is a state of increased awareness. (See Figure 2.1.)

Can a hypnotized person refuse to carry out an instruction from the hypnotist? Absolutely. If I could hypnotize people into doing things they don't want to do, then I'd never stop working because there would be a line to my office and only standing room left. Actually, it's hard enough to hypnotize people to do the things they want to do, such as stopping smoking, letting go of depression, and stopping self-punishment. Hypnosis can make a person 200 times more suggestible than in the waking state, but—and this is a big but—*people have to want to change!* And if the negative feelings and/or beliefs and behaviors are connected to survival in the subconscious, no hypnosis will change the unwanted qualities until the survival connection is changed. That's why subconscious analysis is often needed.

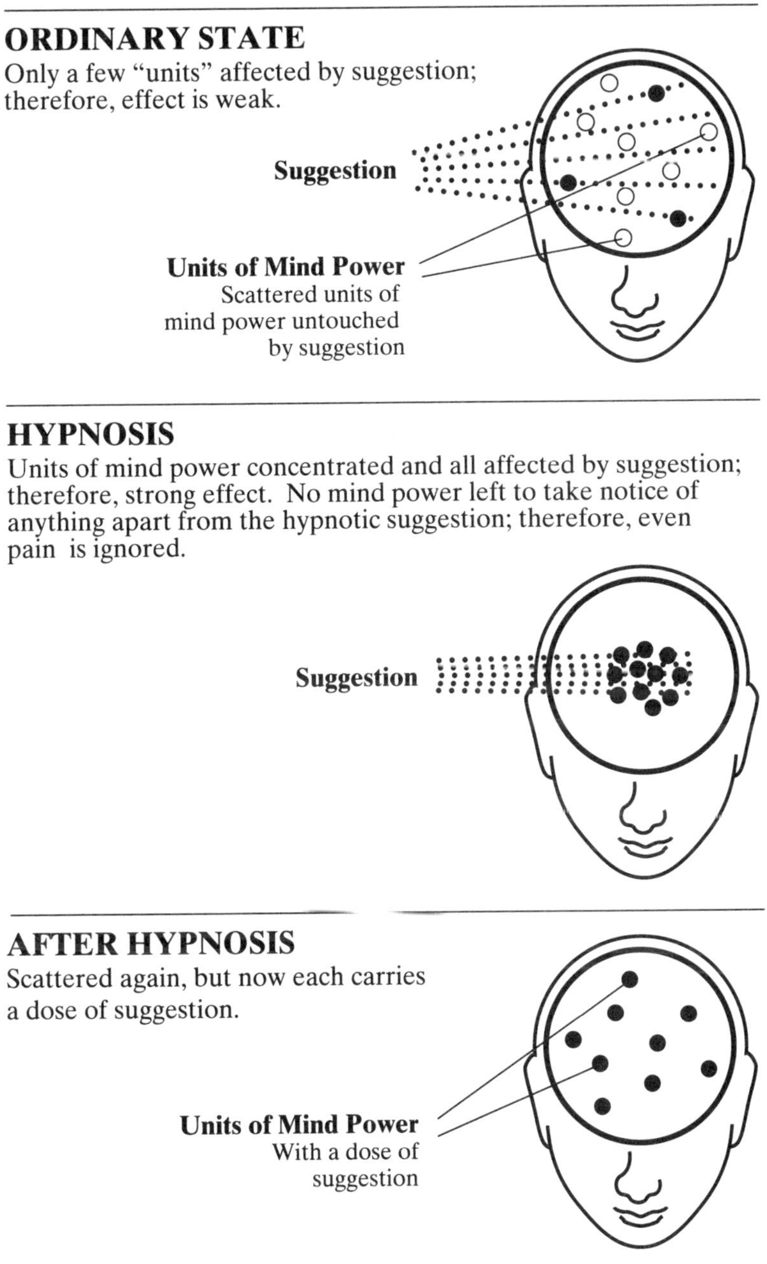

Figure 2.1 Hypnosis is not sleep or unconsciousness, but a superconcentration of the mind. Suggestion is more potent in hypnosis than in ordinary state. (This diagram is an adaptation of the original published in *Modern Hypnotism* by Dr. S. J. Van Pelt, Associated Booksellers, Westport, Connecticut, 1956. Dr. Van Pelt credits the *British Journal of Medical Hypnotism* as the source for the diagram.)

As Dr. Joseph Murphy has pointed out, "A suggestion cannot impose something on the subconscious mind against the will of the conscious mind."[2]

That leads us to the next point. Could a person be persuaded to commit murder while in a state of hypnosis? Yes—if he or she could be persuaded to commit murder under ordinary circumstances. If not, then the answer is "unequivocally no."

MYTHS STILL ABOUND

Hypnosis is not total submission to the caprice of a hypnotist. It is an altered state of consciousness in which the body can be very relaxed and the mind highly focused. We all go through hypnosis at least twice a day. The relaxed state we enter just prior to falling asleep and just prior to waking is a hypnotic state. So is the dreamy feeling you experience on occasion as you take a break from your task and gaze off into the distance.

Suggestions placed in your mind at those times can affect thought and behavior patterns throughout the day as well as program future goals. These two times are optimal times to program your attitude with positive thoughts. People who, after the alarm sounds, lie in bed telling themselves how much they dread the day's activities will have a difficult day. If, by contrast, they tell themselves during that drowsy state that they are getting better and better at what they do, then that day will be a good day. They will feel better, they will approach their day's activities differently, and they will get positive results.

The Encyclopedia Britannica gives the following definition of hypnosis:

> Hypnosis is the term applied to a unique, complex form of unusual but normal behavior which can probably be induced in all normal persons under suitable conditions and also in many persons suffering from various types of abnormality. It is primarily a special psychological state with certain physiological attributes, resembling sleep only superficially and marked by a functioning of the individual at a level of awareness other than the ordinary conscious state. . . . when hypnotized, or in the hypnotic trance, the subject can think, act and behave in relationship to either ideas or reality objects as adequately as, and *usually better than,* he can in the ordinary state of awareness. In all probability this ability derives from intensity and restriction of attention to the task in hand, and the consequent freedom from the ordinary conscious tendency to orient constantly to distracting, even irrelevant, reality considerations.[3] (Emphasis mine.)

William Jennings Bryan, Jr., M.D., the man who introduced hypnoanalysis to many health practitioners and who was instrumental in getting hypnosis accepted by the American Medical Association in 1958, defined hypnosis simply as "a state of superconcentration of the mind."[4]

Baltimore dentist Bruce Goldberg, who maintains practices both in dentistry and hypnotism, defines hypnosis as "a state of increased suggestibility accompanied by a focusing of one's concentration on one thought, idea or person."[5] Goldberg also describes the experience as "simply a way of relaxing and setting aside the conscious mind while at the same time activating the subconscious mind so that suggestions can be made directly to the subconscious, enabling the patient to act on these suggestions with greater ease and efficiency."[6]

Dr. Herbert Spiegel, former Columbia University professor of psychiatry, who is a leading hypnotherapist, describes hypnosis as "a state of aroused intense concentration, *the opposite of sleep*," (emphasis mine) and identifies three types of hypnosis: spontaneous, formal, and self-hypnosis.[7]

Herbert Benson, M.D., author of the best-seller *The Relaxation Response*, defines hypnosis as "an altered state of consciousness which is artificially induced and characterized by increased receptiveness to suggestions."[8]

HYPNOSIS IS NOT A SLEEP STATE

Hypnotized subjects are aware of their surroundings at all times. The mind, however, directs its attention more to the suggestions from the hypnotist than to what is happening in the environment. The hypnotic state is similar to being in a daydream, except that the subject is controlling the daydream, with the hypnoanalyst acting as a guide. It does not mean abdication of personal morals, however. People in hypnosis will do nothing that they would not normally do during any other state of consciousness.

Ernest R. Hilgard, director of Stanford University's Laboratory of Hypnosis Research, shed some light on this fact in an interview in the January 1986 issue of *Psychology Today*. "You don't really do anything that's against your basic value system," Hilgard said. "If you're instructed to do such a thing, you simply come out of hypnosis. For example, if you ask a person to strike someone else with a paper dagger, he'll do it. Give him a real dagger, and he'll drop it."

So much for the movie cliffhangers!

Hilgard also recounted a nineteenth-century experiment in hypnosis. French psychologist Pierre Janet reported that a group of medical students hypnotized a nurse and asked her to take off her clothes. Instantly, she came out of hypnosis. However, one of Hilgard's colleagues tried to recreate the experiment by asking a hypnotized young woman to unbutton her clothes before a group of male students. Much to the colleague's surprise, the woman started to take off her blouse. As it turned out, the woman was a professional stripper. Taking her clothes off in front of an audience was not contrary to her value system; indeed, it was her bread and butter!

In hypnosis, the body can be very relaxed while the mind is superconcentrated and open to acceptable suggestion. The subject remains aware of the environment. Should any major change occur, such as a book dropping or a door slamming, the subject immediately would come out of hypnosis. Barring any dramatic change in the environment, the hypnotized subject focuses attention on the hypnotist's suggestions more than upon other simultaneously occurring phenomena.

However, subjects will not, while in hypnosis, reveal secrets or other information that they would not reveal at any other time. Even in trances required for age regressions, people are capable of making choices. They may witness an event in which they were embarrassed or committed an act that they disapprove of or prefer not to share with the therapist. Unless they subconsciously want to reveal the information, that event remains sealed.

Another common myth about hypnosis is the fear of symptom substitution. Let's say I am using age regression to identify the cause of a person's problem and discover that in the subject's early childhood he or she had an experience that caused a now-undesirable behavior. Once the root cause is discovered, reprogramming suggestions are given to eliminate the problem, not to provide a substitute.

A client came to me recently saying, "I want to quit smoking." That first statement is interesting. She did not say her problem was smoking; she said she wanted to quit smoking.

In Chapter Three, I will discuss the complete procedure I follow when I work with a client. In the following abbreviated case history, my aim is only to illustrate briefly the hypnoanalytic method of getting rid of a particular symptom:

I. H. told me she had not felt particularly loved and accepted by her mother and had started smoking with her girlfriends. When she smoked she felt that she was a part of the gang. The cigarettes made her feel loved and accepted. Obviously, she was mistaking approval for love. She recalled that as a teenager she felt insecure about growing up, and smoked more when she was out with people. She still smoked more in public than when she was alone, indicating that she still was not completely confident around others.

We talked about all these factors; however, she wasn't sure she was ready to quit. I hypnotized her and regressed her back to the first time she smoked. She said:

> I'm in my front yard. My best friend and I are there. We're 16 or 17. We're laughing, like we're getting away with something. This fat boy comes by and laughs at us. He tells us how to inhale. We are totally dizzy.

There was some challenge there, and I. H. recognized that a part of her was rebellious at that time and that being connected to her girlfriends was helpful then but hurtful now.

I gave her suggestions about quitting smoking, stopping her rebellion, feeling alive, and loving herself. She agreed to leave the cigarettes in the past.

At this writing, more than a year and a half has passed and she has not resumed smoking. Often, the mere uncovering of the emotional root of an undesirable behavior is enough to eliminate it.

A BRIEF HISTORY OF HYPNOSIS

Although the term "hypnosis" wasn't coined until 1842, there is evidence that people had practiced the art since before recorded history. The oldest written record of hypnotic treatments dates back to about 3000 B.C. In the Ebers Papyrus, the Egyptians described a treatment in which the physician placed his hands on a patient's head. Professing to have incredible therapeutic powers, the physician uttered strange sounds that reportedly healed the patient. The "sleep temples" of Egypt, Greece, Rome, and Asia Minor actually were hypnotic centers of old.

Hippocrates, the Greek physician known as "the father of medicine," was discussing what we now know as hypnosis when he said, "The afflictions suffered by the body the soul sees quite well with shut eyes." Tenth-century physician Avicenna said, "The imagination can fascinate and modify man's body, either making him ill or restoring him to health."

Franz A. Mesmer introduced hypnotism to the medical profession in the late eighteenth century. Mesmer learned the art from a Catholic priest named Father Gassner, who was an exorcist. From Mesmer's well-known practice came the terms "mesmerism" and "mesmerized." Although Mesmer's healing activity became controversial and his popularity waned with leading medical practitioners at the time, some physicians continued to practice the art.

In 1842, James Braid, a British ophthalmologist, replaced the term "mesmerism" with "hypnotism," after the Greek word *hypnos*, meaning sleep. Although the British Medical Association rejected Braid's offer to read a paper on hypnosis at one of its meetings, Braid, unlike Mesmer, remained in excellent standing in the medical community. When Braid realized years later that hypnotism was not true sleep, he tried in vain to change the name to "mono-ideaism." By that time, however, the words "hypnosis" and "hypnotism" were well entrenched in every European language.

Hypnosis in America was widely associated with charlatans and with stage shows as a form of entertainment until Dr. William Jennings Bryan, Jr., founded the American Institute of Hypnosis in 1955. That was the same year the British Medical Association officially endorsed the teaching of hypnosis in all medical schools. As Bryan reported in "A History of Hypnosis" in the January 1963 issue of *The Journal of the American Institute of Hypnosis*:

> Until that time there had been no educational body devoted exclusively to promoting all the phases of hypnosis in medicine and dentistry, and the Institute was founded to fill that gap. (It) has grown . . . to become the world's most respected educational institution devoted solely to teaching hypnosis . . . to physicians and dentists all over the world.

In 1958, the American Medical Association recognized hypnosis as a legitimate approach to solving certain medical problems. In the three decades since, thousands of operations of all kinds—including open-heart surgeries—have been performed on patients using no anesthesia other than hypnosis.

Many physicians recognize that the mind and body interact to cause illness. They realize that if the mind can create ill health, it also can heal. The mind and body are integrated parts of a whole being; a change in one part affects the others.

Physicians who agree with this philosophy refer patients to professional hypnoanalysts. Hypnoanalysts have backgrounds and training in the basics of developmental psychology, psychopathology, psychotherapy, and, of course, hypnosis.

HYPNOANALYSIS VS. PSYCHOANALYSIS

Hypnoanalysis is analysis of the subconscious mind using hypnosis to identify the origin of a problem and to redirect the energy that had previously been used to sustain the problem toward a solution. Hypnosis opens the door to the subconscious. Analysis provides insight into the cause of the problem, and the hypnoanalyst offers the patient options toward finding a solution.

During the late nineteenth and early twentieth centuries, the medical world more or less shelved hypnosis. Instead, it favored Freudian psychoanalysis. Sigmund Freud was never satisfied with his own results as a hypnotist; he preferred the "free association" technique, or working with responses from fully conscious patients. Maybe Freud was a lousy hypnotist?

As Freud's popularity grew, he denounced hypnosis and the public began to associate the practice solely with direct suggestion. Direct suggestion, however, is only a single aspect of hypnotism. The general public did not understand that the art of hypnotism included both analysis and suggestion.

The goal of therapy with medical hypnoanalysis is to locate and counteract the negative suggestions received in a person's life relating to symptoms and help the individual to drop the defenses that prevent them from maximizing their humanness.

Hypnoanalysis often involves the use of age regression while the patient is in hypnosis to reveal psychologically damaging experiences that have led to some emotional dysfunction that may manifest itself in symptomatic behavior. In hypnosis, the patient can relive the damaging experience to produce an emotional release of the suggestion in the subconscious mind. This process paves the way to recovery. With the origin of the problem uncovered, the hypnoanalyst unties this subconscious knot, freeing the patient to live a healthier, more productive life.

In other words, hypnoanalysis is successful because it goes straight to the subconscious root of the problem. It treats the cause, or the underlying reason, for problems, and not just the symptoms. For example, people physically or psychologically addicted to anything, be it sugar, drugs, alcohol, tobacco, or whatever, usually have a psychologically based underlying reason or reasons for their strong attachments. If allowed to remain unchecked, the passion growing from their addictions could cause physical problems. Likewise, people suffering from intense phobias nearly always discover through analysis that their fears are the result of earlier emotional shocks. All fears except fear of loud noises and falling are learned. People who suffer from various phobias often restrict their activities to avoid the objects or situations of their fears. These avoidances frequently result in emotionally crippling life-styles. Through hypnoanalysis, a person can discover the cause of such fears and overcome them to lead a normal, productive life. Actually, removing fear is one of our easiest operations.

This makes rapid hypnoanalysis a superior method to the tediously slow and often ineffective process of psychoanalysis. While psychoanalysis often lasts as long as five to six years, most, though not all, hypnoanalysis cases last from six weeks to three months.

Another benefit is that, of all medical therapies, hypnosis is the safest. It involves no drugs or surgeries, and it causes no harmful side effects.

Finally, hypnosis feels good; it is beneficial to the body, for relaxation is a precursor to health.

In *The Relaxation Response*, Dr. Benson shows how relaxation is related to good health. Benson first describes the "fight-or-flight" response. This is the body's response to the threat of danger. Notes Benson, "When we are faced with situations that require adjustment of our behavior, an involuntary response increases our blood pressure, heart rate, rate of breathing, blood flow to the muscles, and metabolism, preparing us for conflict or escape."[9]

This response was vital for primitive people contending with physical threats in a wilderness environment. When confronted with a bear or lion, Neanderthals needed the physical energy to swing their clubs effectively or to run for the nearest tree. That kind of behavioral adjustment is rarely called for in modern man; yet our body responds as if our survival did depend upon fighting or fleeing.

"When not used appropriately, which is most of the time, the fight-or-flight response repeatedly elicited may ultimately lead to the dire diseases of heart attack and stroke," writes Benson.[10]

Fortunately, animals, including humans, have developed a physiologic response that counteracts the fight-or-flight response. It's what Benson calls the "relaxation response."

This, he says, is "a natural and innate protective mechanism against 'overstress,' which allows us to turn off harmful bodily effects, to counter the effects of the fight-or-flight response."[11] This response decreases the heart rate, lowers metabolism, decreases the rate of breathing, and brings the body back into a healthier balance.

Hypnosis with suggested deep relaxation can evoke the same physiologic changes as the relaxation response, Benson tells us. It results in decreased oxygen consumption, decreased respiratory rate, and decreased heart rate. Hence, hypnosis can be an important ally in the fight against heart disease and stroke.

GOING TO THE SOURCE

Now that you know more about hypnosis and medical hypnoanalysis, you may be wondering how this may apply to you and your problems. Through hypnosis, you have greater access to the subconscious attitudes and feelings that are responsible for your behavior and/or thoughts. Your hypnoanalyst will be able to uncover the subconscious origin of your problems and can use gentle suggestions to help you remove limiting beliefs and to construct positive, life-affirming attitudes. Through medical hypnoanalytic treatment, you can free yourself to live a healthier, more productive and successful life, whether that success is in an emotional, financial, or spiritual sense.

In later chapters of *Wide Awake, Clear Headed, and Refreshed*. . . , we will discuss such common problems as smoking, weight control, and various phobias and problems that can be successfully treated through medical hypnosis and subconscious analysis. Turn to Chapter Three to find further information on medical hypnoanalysis and a description of the treatment technique I use.

Key Concepts

- Hollywood melodramas are to hypnosis what yellow journalism is to solid news reporting.
- When in hypnosis, one is conscious and more aware of everything that is happening than one is when in the usual state of consciousness.
- Hypnosis is an altered state of consciousness in which the body is very relaxed and the mind is highly focused.
- Everyone goes through hypnosis at least twice a day: The relaxed states we enter just prior to falling asleep and just after waking are hypnotic states. So is the dreamy feeling we experience on occasion as we take a break from our tasks and gaze off into the distance, as well as the state we enter when we're creative, and when time becomes distorted.
- Hypnotized subjects are aware of their surroundings at all times. Their minds, however, direct attention more to the suggestions they receive from the hypnotists than to things that are happening in the environment.
- People in hypnosis will do nothing they would not normally do during any other state of consciousness.
- Although the term "hypnosis" wasn't coined until 1842, there is abundant evidence that people have practiced the art since before recorded history.
- Hypnoanalysis is analysis of the subconscious mind, using hypnosis to identify the origin of a problem and to redirect toward a solution the energy that had previously been used to sustain the problem.
- The goal of therapy with medical hypnoanalysis is to erase the negative suggestions received in a person's life and to help individuals to drop the useless defenses and guarding that prevent them from maximizing their capabilities.

Growth Exercise

1. The next time *Count Dracula* appears on cable TV, watch the scene where Bella Lugosi "hypnotizes" the beautiful woman he desires.
2. Notice times during the day when you get dreamy or time distorts as when you are being creative or really "into" something. These are examples of natural hypnosis.
3. During your presleep state, while dozing off, ask someone to give you suggestions and notice your responses to:
   a. Positive suggestions
   b. Negative suggestions
4. List several areas, qualities, feelings, thoughts, or behaviors you'd like to change in your life?

   ____

   ____

   ____

   ____

WIDE AWAKE, CLEAR HEADED, AND REFRESHED . . .

CHAPTER THREE

REALITY IMPROVEMENT: THE POSSIBLE DREAM

This is the true joy in life, the being used for
a purpose recognized by yourself as a mighty one;
the being a force of nature instead of a feverish,
selfish little clod of ailments and grievances
complaining that the world will not devote
itself to making you happy.

I am of the opinion that my life
belongs to the whole community,
and, as long as I live it is my
privilege to do for it whatever I can.

I want to be thoroughly used up
when I die, for the harder I work
the more I live. I rejoice in life
for its own sake. Life is no "brief
candle" to me. It is a sort of
splendid torch which I have got
hold of for the moment, and I want
to make it burn as brightly as
possible before handing it on to
future generations.

—George Bernard Shaw

AN EFFECTIVE INSTRUMENT FOR HELPING

Hypnoanalysis is an effective wedding of two concepts: Hypnosis and analysis. As an effective instrument for helping people who have problems too difficult to deal with alone, hypnoanalysis should be counted as the weapon of choice.

Hypnoanalysis can lead to permanent positive results for problems such as low self-esteem, depression, guilt, anxieties, and phobias. The analyst helps the patient identify the subconscious beginnings of these problems and nullifies and counteracts their interference with the patient's life.

But not all problems of the mind stem from singular events that trigger depression, anxieties, and phobias. Some of them are rooted in personalities molded by pervasive conditions of upbringing. People who have personality disorders and people who are brought up in dysfunctional, alcoholic, or abusive home situations may need to undergo constructive personality changes. Such changes require fundamental revamping of basic belief systems. There is no more effective theater in our culture for that change to take place than intensive therapy.

In such instances, I usually follow up individual therapy with group sessions before turning the patient loose to work alone, utilizing relaxation and self-hypnosis. Through this integrated system of hypnoanalysis, psychotherapy, and group therapy, people can grow and mature in their own time and in their own ways. Unresolved developmental tasks require more than therapist and client to reach satisfactory conclusions. That's where the groups help.

A word of caution: Though I recommend self-hypnosis to my patients, this technique should not be confused with self-analysis. People sometimes ask, "Why can't I read up on hypnoanalysis and do my own therapy?" Self-help materials often do provide a certain level of knowledge and understanding, but there are limitations to self-analysis.

Hypnoanalysis and psychotherapy are complex disciplines, and the hypnotic tool is just one part of it. No matter how clearly an author may describe principles, ideas, and theories, lay readers may misunderstand, or they may read into the materials the notions that they want. They are apt to miss important points or nuances of self-help ideas. They may unconsciously oversimplify, overlook, or edit the author's ifs, ands, and buts. Many readers of self-help books have entirely misinterpreted the authors' intended results while picking up slogans or buzz words and misapplying them to people and situations.

So while encouraging and utilizing patient self-hypnosis as support for the hypnoanalysis and group-therapy processes, I discourage solo flights. The client needs the concerned objectivity of a therapist to guide the individual toward resolution of the problem at its root.

Through systematic and periodic checking on a patient, a therapist can determine whether the message is getting through and whether the ideas and principles promulgated are being understood and followed.

A TYPICAL SESSION

Medical hypnoanalysis is not scary. Let me describe briefly what happens when a patient comes to my office. Case studies throughout this book will give more insight into the process.

First, I take a history, as they do in the medical profession before embarking on treatment. My initial question is nearly always "What's the problem?" Usually, within the first two or three sentences, the patient will reveal the information that turns out to be related to the basic diagnosis. Before getting into background information, I follow the first question with such queries as "How long has it been a problem?" "What makes it worse?" "What makes it better?" "What could you do if you are cured of this that you cannot do now?" "What will be the result of your treatment?" "What do you expect?"

Answering questions during the history-taking period allows a person to let go. Often, patients have never talked to anyone about some of the issues I ask about. If a patient refuses to answer questions about some areas of his or her past, there may be decreased hope of solving the problem.

I remember a patient who came to see my supervisor when I was in graduate school. Mrs. X had trouble breathing and had to carry an oxygen apparatus wherever she went. In addition to chemotherapy for a cancerous tumor in her chest, hypnoanalysis was recommended. My supervisor explained to the patient that a complete history would be necessary before she could begin hypnoanalysis. Mrs. X agreed reluctantly but refused to answer questions concerning her childhood and adolescence. Actually, she vehemently opposed any discussion of her mental-emotional state and discontinued treatment after a few visits.

Mrs. X's emotional constriction and subsequent depression and unhappiness were apparent. Her tumor, it seems, was related to her mind-set.

Researchers and other clinicians, such as I, see evidence of this connection between mind-set and illness on a daily basis. It's a good bet, however, that she could have been much happier and probably would have been helped if she had opened up the hurt, pain, anger, and resentment she had stored inside. Cancer is, after all, biological suicide.

I don't know what happened to Mrs. X, but I suspect she died not long after that. The tumor, by the way, was lodged next to her heart and threatened its function. I am convinced that her heart was emotionally dead and her mind was attempting to make the mental image a physical reality. She was probably a victim of the spiritual and physical walking-zombie syndrome. A syndrome, in medicine, is a number of symptoms occurring together and characterizing a specific disease. In hypnoanalysis, we also identify certain conditions by a set of symptoms that characterize them. The walking-zombie syndrome is one of them. Later, we will also describe the Ponce de Leon syndrome.

Hypnoanalysis is a nonthreatening procedure. Once I know the reason the patient has come and what his or her hopes and expectations are, our conversation can turn to earlier history with questions on marital status, home life, school, and relationships with parents, with siblings, and with peers.

Following the history, during which we establish some trust and understanding, the patient reclines in a comfortable lounge chair in a private room, wearing a headset and a blindfold while I am in a nearby control room. I gently guide the patient into a state of relaxation.

That essentially is what hypnosis is all about—relaxation. It's a natural state of mind that opens the door to the subconscious. During hypnosis, the patient's conscious awareness retreats and the mind becomes superconcentrated. At this stage, I administer a word-association test, which helps clarify my understanding of the individual's attitudes and feelings, and conclude by giving the patient a suggestion to have a dream about his or her problem. Our word-association tests are based on the work of Dr. William Jennings Bryan, Jr., M.D., and are comparable to the medical doctor's blood tests, urinalysis, or X rays. They help to clarify the issues and support diagnoses.

In subsequent sessions, I discuss with clients their responses to the word-association tests, analyze their dreams, and usually teach them to practice hypnosis.

The dream analysis is a further diagnostic test. It pinpoints the area needing understanding. Often the dream reveals that a patient's problem originated before memory or at birth, and sometimes even in a past life—or at least in what the patient remembers as a past life. The dream is a direct message from the patient's subconscious mind and, therefore, is essential to the analysis.

Usually, by that point in the treatment, the patient is ready to age regress, under hypnosis, back to the beginning of the problem, the initial sensitizing event. (This concept is analogous with surgery in medicine.) By communicating with the subconscious, I am able to uncover the underlying reason behind the patient's problem, addiction, or phobia. Then, in later sessions, we deal with those problems and resolve them. We remove from the subconscious the negative thoughts that cause a person's problem.

Hypnoanalysis is frequently a quick process. It takes about six sessions to help a client stop smoking. Problems such as phobias and depression may take 12 to 20 sessions to resolve. Persons with more serious conditions, such as codependence, sexual abuse, or long-standing personality problems, often choose to follow up in group therapy, supplemented with regular private sessions.

GETTING TO THE ROOT OF THE PROBLEM

I just noted that we often find the roots of patients' problems by following the memory trail. We do so by the process of age regression. In age regression, the patient's memory returns, through hypnosis, to an earlier period in life. This regression can take the individual back to the time of birth, and even to the time before birth, when the patient's only world was the womb.

Where does the trail of memory begin? One of the most fascinating aspects of hypnosis is its ability to draw, from an individual's subconscious, memories that seem to have been born in previous lives. Sometimes, these memories expose the roots of problems plaguing the individual in the present life. John provides an example of past-life regression as one key to solving a long-standing problem.

John came to me at age 65, concerned about a life-long lack of motivation, low energy, and frequent bouts of depression. His wife had died four years earlier. He was interested in past lives and believed in reincarnation. He stated:

> All my life, I've been a loner. I seem content doing nothing. I've had all kinds of businesses and I never really lasted. The problem now is that I am looking at the rest of my life like that. I can't do anything. I sit and watch TV. I can't relate to people, seem to put them off. I've been wondering what makes me tick for some years.

I asked what he thought he could do once he was cured that he could not now do, and he responded, "I think I could start enjoying life just a little bit." This was his subconscious fear: enjoying life.

In our early conversation, John used such phrases as "off-hand." He said his depression was better "in cycles, almost monthly" (like a woman's menstrual cycle). "People can take advantage of me in nothing flat and I let them." He said something about "never really lasting." This sounded as if his problem might have sexual overtones.

I asked him how his sex relations were and he said, "They are nowhere. I haven't had sex in a number of years." His history indicated he was reared in the Catholic faith, had married at 22, and had never had sexual relations with anyone other than his wife.

Since his wife's death, he had been wanting to establish relationships with other people but had found himself unable to do so. "I don't have any friends. I'm amazed, now that I look at it, how I got through life without any friends," he observed. When the question of guilt came up, he said, "I am not the kind of man I wish I were, for my marriage."

When I asked what he wanted from me, he said, "I want to be able to talk to people, have relationships with them, and not to be putting things off all the time."

Part of the word-association test under hypnosis went this way:

Ryan: Problem . . .
John: Solving.
Ryan: Desire . . .
John: A better life.
Ryan: There must be . . .
John: Absolution. (Indicates he feels guilt for some reason.)
Ryan: Not having sex feels like . . .
John: It's a pleasant memory.

We have several terms in the word-association test that are considered slang. They give us a clue to a person's attitude about sexuality, whether they relate to sex from an adult or a childish perspective. In the test, here are those words:

Ryan: Prick . . .
John: Puncture.
Ryan: Pussy . . .
John: Cat.

RYAN: Fuck . . .
JOHN: A four-letter word. (He shook his head.)
RYAN: Cock . . .
JOHN: Rooster.
RYAN: Peter . . .
JOHN: St. Peter.
RYAN: Come . . .
JOHN: Escapes me. (It does escape him, because this is significant.)
RYAN: It all started when . . .
JOHN: I don't know.
RYAN: It got worse when . . .
JOHN: I got married.

I learned two things from those word associations: He relates to sexuality as a child would. His problem (reaching out to people) started earlier, but worsened when he got married. He related to sexuality as a child would—e.g., giving responses such as "cat," "rooster," etc.

The next step in treatment is to analyze a client's dream. John's dream dealt with childhood relationships. "They just made me feel we were poor and there was nothing we could do about it. I was pretty much ignored. I was afraid to relate to people," he said.

That was when the part of John's personality that allowed him to interact with others had died. Under hypnosis, I helped him bring that back to life.

In subsequent sessions, we did a regression to the womb. He had a pretty good experience during that stage, but when advanced to the birth, he said:

> I feel strange. I am crying. It is a short time. Somebody is picking me up. It is real strange being washed off. Back with Mom, it feels good. She is smiling.

It was evident that during his initial environmental experience (IEE, a term that will creep up repeatedly in this book), his earliest experience with someone other than his mother, someone had given him a feeling of being strange. He had identified this as the appropriate feeling when relating to people.

I helped John understand that this feeling had probably programmed him to feel strange with people. He agreed that his reaction to strangers was inappropriate and was willing to abandon it. In another regression, I brought him back to a time when he was in his mother's arms, crying. Somebody, a stranger, was attempting to take a picture of him in tears, and he felt very bad about it.

I removed his negative feelings concerning those incidents, and for the first time since the beginning of his treatment (about eight sessions), positive change became evident. He came into his next session saying, "Well, I have a tremendous amount of energy. I don't know where to put it." (Think of this in a literal way).

He wanted to be regressed to a past life during which he indicated that he had some image about a rape scene. This is how he described the scene:

> I am walking through clouds or fog. Above the ground. There is green grass and green trees. A red barn. An open door. Some kind of shoes, leather, ankle high. Black stockings, horse and buggy inside. Nothing in there.
>
> Back on the road again. Concrete, white, dirty. People are there. An old woman. I am about 8 or 10 years old. Inside a building. Climbing up steps. A room or window without glass . . . like I am aimless.

Then he switched to another scene:

> I am riding on a horse. I am male. It is very dark. It is almost like a picture of Rome. There are robes. I seem to be going down a hill, a rocky hill. There is just nothing.

In these two lifetimes, the feeling that he described as relating to the here and now, was a feeling of being empty, of being aimless, of not really existing. Not having any connection to the world.

I helped him put those feelings in the past and gave him positive suggestions to be connected to this life. He let go of the negativity he had carried over from those existences and adopted instead positive suggestions about getting involved with people.

An interesting subsequent regression proved to be even more productive. I regressed John to the womb once more because he still seemed to experience difficulty in establishing personal relationships. Suddenly, as he was describing typical contented feelings inside the womb, he jumped to a past life, saying he felt as if he had been there long enough, as if he were running. He began reporting what he saw in an excited voice, staccato fashion:

> I'm on the side of a hill, running away. It is a person . . . the feeling I have had all my life . . . like holding my breath. (He sounded frightened.)
>
> Somebody is running after me. I seem to be on a shore. There is a sailing ship there. A harbor. I am always so damned curious. I've got to find out what is on the ship.

> I go up the gangplank of the ship. I am very tense. Visions of a body here and a body there. Looks like foul play. It's somebody's big, long knife. A sabre. A pirate. He is very menacing.
>
> I turn tail and take off like a bullet. I am slowed down to a walk and I still have this feeling, this fear.

John felt his life was in danger. While he was still under hypnosis, I helped him to leave those fears in the past life, to recognize that his life now was not in danger.

I saw John only two more times, but he reported two years later that he was doing very well. His early environmental experiences involving others and several past lives he produced spontaneously had programmed his lack of motivation and his inability to develop meaningful relationships. After hypnoanalysis, he began dating women and having sexual relations.

Whether the past-life information is real or not is immaterial. We could consider it a manifestation—a metaphor—of what is happening in John's subconscious mind. And that's primarily how I treat material such as this.

With that framework to go on, accepting what John came up with and removing the negative suggestions he had received in his subconscious mind—wherever they came from—I was able to cure him of his problem in about 15 sessions. That is a relatively short treatment time, considering the lengthy periods of time involved in many other therapy approaches. Having practiced several other approaches, I personally can attest to the relative rapidity with which hypnoanalysis resolves many problems.

HYPNOSIS IS A VEHICLE

Hypnosis is a tool. Anyone can learn hypnotic techniques. An astute 10-year-old can learn to be a hypnotist. The hard part to the hypnoanalytic process is the subconscious analysis—helping people pull out the negative suggestions from their subconscious minds, nullifying them and providing reeducation and rehabilitation through positive suggestions. Remember, the patient under hypnosis always remains in control. Hypnosis involves cooperation from the subject; no trance can be imposed on someone against hes or her will. The subject who actively resists the hypnotist's suggestions will be about as hypnotizable as a brick. (How many hypnoanalysts does it take to change a light bulb? Only one, but the light bulb must want to change.)

Therein lies a basic truth about hypnotism. Since the subject must cooperate to reach a state of hypnosis, it means that all hypnosis is self-hypnosis.

The subject willingly enters the altered state of consciousness. This also means that all of us can achieve self-hypnosis—without the aid of a hypnotist—and program our minds for improved functioning. Most of us do it all the time. We will see how shortly.

As a result of hypnosis, we can develop greater access to subconscious attitudes and feelings that are responsible for our behaviors. Serious problems, addictions, and phobias require help from licensed professionals. However, through self-hypnosis, you can feed yourself gentle suggestions to help remove restrictive, self-confining beliefs and replace them with positive, life-affirming values.

YOUR TWO BRAINS

Before we go into a deeper discussion of hypnotism, let's take a look at the part of you where hypnosis takes place: your brain.

Scientists have known for a long time that the brain is divided into two hemispheres. They refer to them as the left brain and the right brain.

You spend most of your time thinking with your left brain. You use your left hemisphere when you talk, read, balance your checkbook, and figure your income tax. The left side of the brain is the logical side. You use it to reason.

But reasoning isn't the only aspect of mental activity. Some of mankind's greatest discoveries have come through insight and intuition. Somehow, the brain takes a "short cut" to knowledge and understanding. This "short cut" involves the right hemisphere.

The right brain is the source of your ideas, intuition, imagination, and emotions. It houses your spatial sense, your musical abilities, and your ability to image. Symphonies are composed, poems are written, great paintings are created, and hunches are born in the right brain. When you see a familiar face, your right brain recognizes it. Your left brain supplies the name that goes with the face. You are at the peak of your mental powers when your left brain and your right brain are in balance.

At any given time, you are functioning at one of four mental-activity levels. These levels are defined by the frequency of electrical waves produced by the brain and measured on an electroencephalograph. They are as follows:

1. Beta level. You function at the beta level—the level of complete consciousness—most of your waking hours. In this state, the brain's electrical waves are pulsing at a rate of more than 14 cycles per second. It's in the beta state that you complete most routine activities. Both the subconscious and conscious minds are functioning, and concentration efficiency is about 25 percent at this level.

2. Alpha level. Alpha waves tend to have the highest voltages of all brain waves, and they usually are measured at 8 to 13 cycles per second. Alpha waves tend to be produced when an adult person is relaxed and awake, but with eyes closed.[1] This is the level where hypnosis occurs. Concentration efficiency is at 95 percent to 100 percent. Individuals in the alpha state will be relaxed and their limbs will feel heavy, but their bodies' senses will be acute. Typical activities on this level, in addition to hypnosis, are daydreaming, meditation, going into natural sleep, or awaking.

3. Theta level. Deep hypnosis and light sleep are typical of the theta level, when the brain is emitting waves at four to seven cycles per second. They appear in the deepest meditation of some Zen masters. Dr. Barbara Brown of Sepulveda, California, one of the leading researchers in this field, says the theta state seems to be related to "problem-solving, sorting and filing of incoming data, and retrieval of information already deposited in the brain's memory."[2]

4. Delta level. The mind is almost totally at rest at the delta or deep-sleep level, when brain waves have slowed to below four cycles per second. The average adult achieves this brain-activity level for only 30 minutes to an hour each night.

As we've seen, the slow frequencies are the ones that take us into states of relaxation, deep inward focus, and sleep. These states can be induced by mimicking the brain-wave frequencies with pulsed lights, sounds, and electrical current. When brain rhythms follow the rhythms of the stimulation, we call it "entrainment."

Entrainment is the process through which people can be lulled to sleep by the rhythmic crashing of waves against a shore, by the soothing rhythm of a lullabye, and even by the rhythmic clackety-clack of train wheels heard from a Pullman's berth. In my practice, I use a hemispherical synchronization machine to produce entrainment and to help the patient to achieve a hypnotic trance.

During these states, the right brain is ready to receive and remember information, to imagine, and to create. In these states, it is most receptive to suggestion through hypnosis.

WE HYPNOTIZE OURSELVES DAILY

Chances are that you've hypnotized yourself many times without even being aware of it. Have you ever gone to bed knowing that it was important for you to awake at a certain time? Were you surprised the next morning when you awoke, precisely at the desired time, either without an alarm clock or perhaps a minute before the alarm activated? Was it magic? No. It was hypnosis—self-hypnosis. You programmed your subconscious, and it did what it does best: It obeyed your command.

Hypnosis is a state of relaxation that opens the subconscious mind to direct suggestion. As we said earlier, everyone experiences a state of hypnosis at least twice daily—once before awaking and once before falling asleep. At each point, the conscious mind is losing energy, which allows the subconscious to accept the energy and open up to suggestion. That is what happens when you program yourself to wake up at a certain time.

SO IF YOU CAN SLEEP, YOU CAN BE HYPNOTIZED! And remember, a person who is determined not to be hypnotized will not be. By the same token, anyone who is willing to cooperate with a hypnotist—or to practice seriously the principles of self-hypnosis, which we will discuss later—can achieve a hypnotic state at will. By the way, there's a myth that says only people of low intelligence can be hypnotized. People of above-average intelligence actually make the best subjects. Why? Because for intelligence to function, there has to be imagination, and guess what: Imagination is the key to the subconscious.

THE LIGHT HYPNOTIC TRANCE

Within the alpha-theta mind-activity level, hypnosis occurs on three different planes or trances: light, medium, or somnambulistic. Hypnosis begins with a light trance, or focusing of attention, similar to the focusing that occurs when you're involved in an interesting project, engaged in a pleasant daydream, watching an entertaining motion picture, or reading a stimulating book. The conscious mind loses track of time and awareness of environment as it focuses totally on the subject or task at hand. Have you ever driven a car from one city to another, only to realize after reaching your destination that you had little or no memory of the area in between? The reason you didn't remember was that you were lost in thought about another matter unrelated to driving. Your mind was focused, and you were in a light trance—a state of hypnosis. Through repeated experience and conditioning, your subconscious had become conditioned to operate the car with very little conscious thought.

If you are in a trance while watching an interesting movie, then it is only natural that you are open to suggestion. Documented events back up this fact. During the 1930s, for example, Clark Gable took off his shirt in the motion picture *It Happened One Night*, revealing that he wasn't wearing an undershirt. Instantly, undershirt sales plummeted across the country. What a suggestion!

Were people hypnotized into not buying undershirts? A skeptic might maintain that audience members had a strong desire to identify with Clark Gable. But Gable hasn't been around for many years now, and motion-picture producers still charge big bucks to display brand-name products on the screen. It's a subtle form of advertisement that can pay off handsomely. For example, sales of the Reese's Pieces candy skyrocketed after little Elliot fed them to the extraterrestrial being in the blockbuster motion picture *E.T.* People can be entranced by the screen, and while they're entranced their subconsciouses are receptive to suggestions, including suggestions that they buy certain commercial products over others.

Make no mistake: Hypnosis is as powerful as it is simple. As I mentioned in a previous chapter, you can recall popular radio and television commercials years after they cease to be aired. The product jingles or slogans have been instilled into your subconscious mind through the power of repetition. It's no coincidence that the best-selling products are usually the ones that are advertised most often. Advertising is a common form of mass hypnosis for which corporations pay dearly. Returns are virtually assured if the product is any good at all. Hence, advertising abounds.

Why else do you suppose fast-food chains have prospered over the years? The light-trance level, however, is limited in efficiency for age regression and other purposes of medical hypnoanalysts.

THE OPTIMAL MEDIUM-TRANCE LEVEL

Most hypnoanalysts prefer to work at the medium-trance level. On this second plane, an individual is deeply relaxed and more receptive to suggestions. Extraneous noises or activity usually will not break their concentration. The hypnoanalyst has greater access to the client's subconscious mind and can help the individual replace existing attitudes and feelings that are responsible for undesired behaviors.

Age regression can be achieved more satisfactorily at this level. In a medium trance, people may actually relive events that occurred at earlier times. They will experience the physical or emotional pains associated with the events and will probably even adopt the voice quality and vocabulary they possessed when the events occurred—in other words, they will experience a hallucination.

We'll go into greater depth on age regressions in a later chapter, but let me share one of my favorite cases here. I particularly like this case because it demonstrates both age and past-life regression, and points out the tremendous changes a person can make once the root of a problem is exposed.

Depression Was the Symptom Here

A 38-year-old woman came to me in February complaining of depression. She said she was working a lot but had begun to experience exaggerated feelings of loneliness when she was in her apartment. "I could be dead in my apartment and nobody would know," she said. "I'm just feeling alone a lot."

When I asked how long she had had the problem, she said since around the holiday time. I said, "What makes it worse?" and she answered, "Well, seeing a family bothers me. I want one of my own. It just doesn't feel like that's open to me."

I asked, "What makes it better?" and she replied, "Sometimes getting together with people." I asked, "What have you done to help yourself already?" and she responded that she mostly ignored it. "I want to hibernate. . . . Pull in some."

I next asked, "What could you do once you're cured of this feeling that you can't do now?" She replied, "I kind of feel like my life is on hold. I don't know how to answer that." Then she looked upward, as if to heaven, and added, "Having a home feeling, feeling like I belong somewhere most of the time."

With only a page and a half of her history taken, I observed that already this client was saying that she didn't belong. It wasn't just a situational thing; it had to do with her whole feeling about herself belonging in the world.

I asked if she was divorced and whether she was happy. She said, "No, I want to have a home and family and share my life with somebody."

I moved on to questions about school life and learned that she went to college for two years. "Were you happy?" I asked. Her response: "No. I just didn't seem to fit in socially."

I backed up further: "As a child, were you ever so sick that your parents were really concerned about you?" She said, "Up to five, I was anemic. I looked like a walking ghost." When I asked her what her childhood was like, she said, "I'd rather skip it."

I asked her the name of her mother. She told me, so I asked what kind of person her mother was. She said, "I don't know, I never met her." That's when I learned she was given up for adoption.

I asked a second time what she was like as a kid. This time, she said, "Quiet. I read a lot and played by myself."

I concluded the history period by asking what she wanted from me and she said, "I want to get myself back on track. I've slipped a little bit, lately—my motivation. That old 'I don't care' attitude has been slipping in lately."

Some interesting things came out in her word-association test under light hypnosis. I'll recount it as it occurred, staccato fashion:

Ryan: Complete a sentence beginning with the word "who."
Patient: Who am I?
Ryan: Unwanted . . .
Patient: Me.
Ryan: (I said her first name.)
Patient: Me.
Ryan: The real problem . . .
Patient: Me.
Ryan: Life . . .
Patient: Death.
Ryan: Death . . .
Patient: Life.
Ryan: Sin . . .
Patient: Death.

Being "on hold" was the way that she described her life and it was like death to her.

Ryan: If I ever really let go . . .
Patient: I'll die, if I don't get out, I'll die.
Ryan: Underneath it all . . .
Patient: Scared.

RYAN: I'm afraid when . . .
PATIENT: I'm alone.
RYAN: All my life . . .
PATIENT: I wanted to be happy.
RYAN: The one thing I need most is . . .
PATIENT: Love.
RYAN: It all started when . . .
PATIENT: I was born.
RYAN: It got worse, when . . .
PATIENT: I was a teen.

It was clear here that she had a very empty feeling about herself, about her identity. She said it had started when she was born.

RYAN: Guilt . . .
PATIENT: Anger.
RYAN: Punishment . . .
PATIENT: Fine.
RYAN: I punish myself because . . .
PATIENT: I deserve it.
RYAN: My punishment is . . .
PATIENT: Hate.

So she was hating herself. For some reason or another, she got the idea that she hated herself and that she deserved to be punished. This was clearly an identity problem. She was suffering from the spiritual walking-zombie syndrome, which is characterized by loss of self-love, adoption of a guilty feeling, and the tendency to punish oneself.

We reviewed her history and word-association test, and I explained the identity problem and the fact that part of her problem was that she felt like a little girl (Ponce de Leon syndrome). People experiencing the Ponce de Leon syndrome exhibit immature behavior. They do not want to grow up and be responsible for themselves. She agreed with that assessment.

In a subsequent session, I regressed her to the period when she was being carried in the womb. At two months after conception, she said:

> I can't breathe. My chest is heavy. She doesn't want to take care of a baby.

These were thoughts she had received from her mother while she was in the womb.

Then, I regressed her to one week after conception, when her mother was unaware of the pregnancy and had not developed anxiety feelings about having a baby. The patient was then able to feel at peace, happy, as if she belonged in the world.

I led her to remove the negative thoughts that she had taken in from her mother and to bring back to the here and now the feelings of peace, calmness, and tranquility—the feeling of being connected with God, the universe, and everybody in it.

After that, we age progressed month by month finding out what happened when she was in the womb. At four months, she said:

> Something is sitting on my chest. I'm scared.

Then, she described her mother:

> She doesn't like where she is living. She doesn't like my grandparents.

Suddenly, her breathing became real labored. I said, "What's happening?" All of a sudden she said excitedly:

> I'm in a room. It's dark. I'm by myself. I'm in a bed. I'm a little girl. I'm four years old. I'm sick. I've got pneumonia. I'm hurting. It's hot. I die. There is nobody there.

Then, she simply described floating through the clouds.

After she had gone through this experience (a spontaneous past-life regression), which was very emotional, I asked if this was she.

She said, "Yes, but I was in a previous life."

She had been viewing herself at four months past conception when the spontaneous past-life regression occurred. It was directly related to the feeling of something sitting on her chest; the feeling in her chest was from dying of pneumonia. I brought her back to the present, removing negative thoughts and feelings that she carried with her from her earliest experience and the past-life experience.

This spontaneous past-life regression was an unusual event and brings up the issue of reincarnation. The jump occurred because the initial sensitizing event that was causing her to feel a sense of dread and deadness had occurred in that life. I removed those feelings, along with the thoughts and feelings that she had picked up from her mother prior to birth in this life. (Sometimes the phenomenon of age regression results in inaccurate time sequences.)

In a later hypnotic session, we returned to the womb again and brought her to the birth experience. She agitatedly described hurting and said:

> Someone is squeezing me. It doesn't feel good. I want out. I will never get out of here.

The difficult birth experience had conditioned her to feel like change was negative and that she could not make her life work. Stuck! She tied those feelings to what was happening in her here-and-now life, so I asked her to leave those feelings in the past, and she agreed.

From that point, the patient's attitude began to change. She reported being rid of her loneliness and depression and decided to work on another problem through hypnoanalysis. She weighed 155 pounds.

Here's the core of her word-association test on weight:

Ryan: Guilt . . .
Patient: Food.
Ryan: People of the opposite sex consider me . . .
Patient: Ugly.
Ryan: I punish myself because . . .
Patient: I'm ugly.
Ryan: My punishment is . . .
Patient: Being fat.
Ryan: As long as I'm fat, I can avoid . . .
Patient: Men.
Ryan: To me, God is . . .
Patient: Life.
Ryan: To me, food is . . .
Patient: Life.

From the above, I concluded that, in her subconscious mind, food and God were connected.[3] One of the things hypnoanalysts stress in treating the spiritually depressed is that God is love. And love was what she really needed.[4]

Dr. Daniel Zelling once said, "When the spirit is hungry, the body gets fed."

I pointed out to her under hypnosis that she was afraid of men and that when she was scared she turned to food. We did a regression back to her early childhood when she was conditioned to feel that food was love. After the regression, she was able to lose weight, dropping to 120 pounds. This case was a complete success. She turned her life around and is a working professional confronting life without depression or obesity.

SOMNAMBULISTIC TRANCES ARE RARELY USED

Although the third, or somnambulistic, trance is at a very deep level and individuals are more open to suggestion in this state, they still will not break their personal moral codes. Entertainers prefer to work with subjects on this level because a somnambulistic trance usually results in hypnoamnesia. Upon awaking from a trance of this level, individuals may not remember their actions unless they're told to do so. It's in this state also that subjects see objects that are not present (positive hallucinations) or fail to see things that are there (negative hallucinations).

These characteristics make this state ideal for comedy. Only a small percentage of the population can truly achieve a somnambulistic trance, so many of the eager audience participants you see in stage shows are hams who want to be part of the show.

WHY USE HYPNOSIS?

A hypnoanalyst uses hypnosis as a tool to age regress a patient to the event in the subconscious at which an emotional problem originated. At that point, the easy part is over; the rest of the process involves analysis and removal of the problem. That's where the real work is involved. The hypnosis itself is simple—so simple, as I pointed out, that you have probably hypnotized yourself regularly throughout your life.

As a social worker who has practiced traditional psychotherapy, I am more impressed with the rapid results my patients now get through hypnoanalysis. The most intricate of problems can be treated in 30 sessions or fewer with medical hypnoanalysis. When I discovered that hypnoanalysis shifted psychotherapy into "high gear," bringing new impetus and creating solutions in the short term, I was really excited. Through hypnoanalysis, many problems are resolved in six to eight weeks. At last, I can help people quickly, permanently, and successfully.

Hypnoanalysis is analysis of the subconscious mind using hypnosis, a natural state of mind, to identify the origin of a problem and to take the energy that had previously sustained the problem and direct it toward a solution. Hypnosis opens the door to the subconscious; analysis opens understanding to the cause of the problem; and patient and therapist together open up options toward solutions.

As Dr. Bryan pointed out in his taped training sessions, our purpose is to shell out the negative thought and leave the rest of the mind alone. The goal of the hypnoanalyst is to help patients get over the problems that brought them to us, not to treat every little idea and review everything that has happened in their lives. Patients may want to keep some of their hang-ups. That is why, in the initial interview, I require answers to such questions as "What is the problem?" "What do you expect of me?" "What can you do if you are cured of this problem that you cannot do now?"

When positively or negatively influenced suggestions reach the subconscious, the subconscious doesn't discriminate. Negative behavior and attitudes are acquired through negative hypnosis or a negative-focused state of attention resulting from anger, worry, guilt, negative self-talk, and especially fear. Fear causes what you're afraid of to come into existence. Positive attitudes and behavior are the result of positive suggestions or a focused state of attention growing out of productive behavior reinforced by reward, loving attitudes, and positive self-talk.

Medical hypnoanalysis is successful because it goes to the root of a problem. It treats the negative suggestion—the underlying reason for the problem—and not the symptom or the problem itself. Hypnosis gives greater access to subconscious power, allowing replacement of existing attitudes and feelings that are responsible for undesired behaviors, feelings, or physical conditions. The mind becomes more porous under hypnosis. Suggestions that might be repelled during full consciousness can be absorbed while in a hypnotic state. The hypnotic state creates 200 times more suggestibility than is present during the waking state.

WE GET WHAT WE EXPECT

As we learn more and more about the power of the subconscious mind, we can begin to see how hypnoanalysis can improve the quality of our lives, both physically and emotionally. Our subconscious controls our lives and our well-being, our health, and our habits. The key is to accept the fact that we are in control and use that strength to determine our direction. Many people have trouble accepting responsibility for their lives. They prefer to abdicate that responsibility to others, to government, or to God.

Smart physicians have known for centuries that good medical practice does not treat the body and ignore the mind. Hypnosis puts the power of the subconscious to work. Dr. Bryan recounted a controlled experiment in which amphetamines were given to members of one group and barbiturates were given to members of another. Participants of each group were told they received the opposite drug, and they reacted the way they were led to believe they would react, proving that the power of the subconscious is stronger than drugs.[5]

G. Alan Marlatt of the University of Washington and Damaris J. Rohsenow of the V.A. Medical Center in Providence, Rhode Island, substantiated that finding in more recent research. They divided groups of subjects according to whether they expected to receive a vodka and tonic or simply tonic. The results: Expectations affected behavior more than did than the effects of alcohol or the absence of alcohol.

"What the people expected—tonic, or vodka and tonic—determined how aggressively they behaved and how socially anxious and sexually aroused they became," the study found. The drinkers got what they expected, in other words.[6]

Dr. Deepak Chopra, who wrote *Quantum Healing: Exploring the Frontiers of Mind/Body Medicine*, confirms the influence of mind over body:

> The mind is not just confined to your brain. It's in every cell of your body . . . our emotions, our feelings, our desires have a very important role to play in how we respond to disease. . . . About 80 percent of all the drugs that we use in Western medicine are "optional" or of marginal benefit, which means that if we didn't use them, it wouldn't make a bit of difference to the person except save money and prevent side effects.[7]

Chopra says that our bodies manufacture their own anticancer drugs, tranquilizers, and antibiotics; but when we are sad, angry, or under stress, we interfere with our internal pharmacy.[8] According to the former chief of staff of New England Memorial Hospital in Stoneham, Massachusetts, the key to most cures is to get to the basic cause of the disease:

> Technology is very useful and some of the miracles of modern medicine are very remarkable, but we've got to be selective. . . . We have the idea in the USA that there is a pill for everything. If you can't believe you ate the whole thing, then have a couple of Alka Seltzers. If you can't go to sleep, take a sleeping pill. If you're feeling anxious, take a tranquilizer. . . . It's merely treating the symptoms.
>
> . . . The reason people get ill is something very simple: how they think, how they interact with their environment, how they behave and what they eat. . . . Quantum healing simply means understanding the mind-body connection at a deep level and recognizing that if we can act at that level, then we can generate the healing response from within the body itself.[9]

As we move into successive chapters, you will see how you can benefit from hypnosis to replace bad habits with good ones, strengthen good habits, conquer fears and phobias, succeed in any given endeavor, improve your attitudes, and increase your creativity.

Key Concepts

- Medical hypnoanalysis always begins with the taking of a complete patient history.
- Within the first two or three sentences of the history, a patient may reveal information that often turns out to be related to the basic diagnosis.
- If one refuses to answer questions about some areas of one's past, there is a diminution of hope in solving one's problem.
- The history taking helps to establish trust and understanding between patient and hypnoanalyst.
- By communicating with the subconscious, hypnoanalysts are able to uncover the underlying reason behind a patient's problem, addiction, or phobia.
- People of above-average intelligence make the best hypnotic subjects.
- At any given time, we are functioning at one of four mental-activity levels: beta, alpha, theta, or delta.
- Within the alpha-theta mind activity level, hypnosis occurs on three different planes or trances: light, medium, or somnambulistic.
- Most hypnoanalysts prefer to work at the medium-trance level.
- The hypnoanalyst's goal is equal to the patient's goal not to treat every little idea and review everything that happened in their lives.
- Medical hypnoanalysis is successful because it treats the underlying reason for the problem, and not only symptoms.
- We subconsciously control our lives and our well-being, our health, and our habits. The key is to accept that we are in control and use that strength to determine our direction.
- Our bodies manufacture their own anticancer drugs, tranquilizers, and antibiotics; but when we are sad, angry, or under stress, we interfere with our internal pharmacies.

Growth Exercise

1. In three sentences or less, state your problem, or, if more than one problem, use three sentences for each. ______________________________

   ____

   ____

   ____

2. While being honest with yourself, if questioned about your history, are there areas you'd prefer not to divulge? ______________________________

   ____

3. Are those areas related to your problems as far as you know? ________

4. Experiment and learn to identify your brain-wave levels. The goal is to know your most suggestible times.

CHAPTER FOUR

HABITS MAKE LIFE HEAVEN OR HELL

The chains of habit
are generally
too small to be felt
till they are too strong
to be broken.

—*Samuel Johnson*

IT'S YOUR CHOICE

Samuel Johnson was not entirely right. Neither was Horace Mann when he said, "Habit is a cable. We weave a thread of it every day until we cannot break it." Habits are learned behavior. We do establish them by repeated action, but they can be broken.

Habits, both good and bad, are products of our mental conditioning: They result when our subconscious minds accept suggestions. In other words, habits stem from hypnosis, self-hypnosis, or self-suggestion. These suggestions, lodged in our subconscious minds, are there because we decided actively or passively to accept them. We can also decide to dislodge them.

Self-suggestion, or autohypnosis, results in positive or negative purposes. Smokers have hypnotized themselves to believe that cigarettes help them cope with life. Reformed smokers have dehypnotized themselves—or removed the negative suggestion, I should say—to associate cigarettes with reality—death. Chronic overeaters have hypnotized themselves to associate food with love, security, and contentment. Breaking the pattern calls for a new trance, but with a different type of self-suggestion.

Hypnosis is neutral, as is the subconscious mind. The way we program our minds is what makes the difference between heaven or hell. The philosophy among hypnoanalysts is that the key that locked the mind must be used to unlock it. In other words, to be cured, the individual must remove the emotional incident(s) that caused the problem, understand the negative reinforcing behavior and thoughts, and accept positive suggestions to replace the unwanted habits.

Medical hypnoanalysis accomplishes this task incredibly well. Before we look at how we can dislodge unwanted habits, let's consider how we get them in the first place.

IT'S UP TO YOU

Developing a habit is a matter of attitude. Unless physical dependency is involved, most behaviors do not become ingrained overnight. Once a person either accepts or rejects a particular behavior, the seeds are sown. They grow into habits through continued cultivation.

Charles Reade, a nineteenth-century philosopher, said, "Sow an act, and you reap a habit. Sow a habit, and you reap a character. Sow a character, and you reap a destiny."

The path most of us take in developing our character passes three mileposts: Attitudes lead to actions, actions lead to habits, and habits lead to life-styles. Let's look at those steps individually:

1. Attitudes lead to actions. Your thoughts are products of your attitudes. When you feel good about yourself, you tend to function within a positive cycle. You think constructive, productive, healthy thoughts, and your behavior reflects your positive attitude. Conversely, negative attitudes lead to destructive, unproductive, unhealthy thoughts and behavior—a negative, self-limiting cycle.

2. Actions lead to habits. Most of your behavior is based on what makes you feel good or pleasurable. If that's the case, we may ask, why do so many people adopt self-destructive actions? Regardless of how the "more rational" of us look at other people's various destructive behaviors, we have to realize that they are getting some kind of positive rewards from the act or they would not be doing it. The reward can be the avoidance of pain. Nonsmokers may wonder why their smoking friends persist in their habits in spite of the hacking coughs and other consequences that result. Smokers will explain that they like to smoke. It gives them something to do with their hands in social settings. Nondrinkers may wonder why alcohol abusers continue to drink when the practice makes them foolish, dangerous, and hung over. Drinkers will tell you a cocktail (or several) helps them relax. People who shun drugs may wonder why marijuana users persist in assaulting their lungs and numbing their brains. Pot smokers may say that a joint helps them to understand "the real meaning of life."

Frequently, the subconscious reasons for the various destructive habits are hidden from the individual and connected to the person's survival hierarchy. That's where hypnoanalysis and age regression can help. We will go into that later.

3. Habits lead to life-styles. We are a composite of our habits. *Webster's New Collegiate Dictionary* defines a habit as "the prevailing disposition or character of a person's thoughts and feelings: mental makeup."[1] Through internal communication within our conscious minds, our attitudes dictate our actions. Through communication from our conscious to our subconscious minds, our actions dictate our habits. And through communication from our subconscious to our conscious minds, our habits dictate our life-style.

For thousands of years, habits—both forming them and kicking them—have been a matter of concern for philosophers, teachers, parents, politicians, and others concerned with human well-being or human manipulation.

Contrary to what Reade implied, however, our destiny does not have to depend on a pattern of ingrained personal habits. Medical hypnoanalysis offers an alternate route. The practice has come of age in helping us lick unwanted or destructive behavior. One goal of hypnoanalysis is to assist individuals in understanding the basis of their behavior through hypnotic regressions so that they can recognize and deal with their mysterious compulsions and lead happier lives. Once you understand that you didn't set up the rules and values for your life and take responsibility for changing the ones that don't work, then happiness is within your reach.

Hypnoanalysis helps in determining the origin of a habit, a thought pattern, or an area of concern because it allows access to regions of the mind that are not normally accessible. The process is successful because it goes to the root of the problem. It treats the underlying reason for the condition, not the symptom. If you bite your nails, it's not because of a physical addiction you cannot overcome. You bite your nails because of an emotional attachment, a release of tension, etc. If you're a smoker, the real reason for your habit is buried within your subconscious mind, and a successful way to uncover that reason is to communicate with your subconscious. Through hypnosis, you can pull out the reason behind the smoking and then deal with it permanently. Once that is done, you will no longer feel the need to smoke and will need only to concern yourself with the physical dependence, which pales in comparison with the emotional dependence.

Hypnosis gives us greater access to the subconscious attitudes and feelings that are responsible for behavior. A hypnoanalyst can guide a person toward improving behavior and correcting weaknesses by using gentle suggestions to help remove limiting beliefs and to construct positive, life-affirming ones.

The key to success, however, is the patient's desire to change. Hypnoanalysis will work only if an individual wants it to work.

TRIPLE ALLERGENIC THEORY

Dr. Bryan used the "triple allergenic theory," borrowed from medicine, to help identify and understand the development of habits and psychological problems. Bryan theorized that psychological injuries parallel the development of physical allergies. "You can't be allergic to strawberries without eating a strawberry," he pointed out. "You've got to come into contact with a foreign-body protein, an antigen, before the body builds up antibodies against it. . . . The antibodies sit and wait for the antigen to come back again. On the next contact the antigen-antibody action causes the nose to swell or the skin to break out in a rash. The next time you eat strawberries, there are so many antibodies that you get a real big reaction."[2]

The same thing occurs psychologically, Bryan contends. People are born with only two fears: the fear of falling and the fear of loud noises. Think about it. We don't develop a fear of dogs unless we are told to be afraid or unless a dog bites us. A kid would pick up a worm and eat it unless the mother said, "Ugh! That's a worm! Dirty!" The kid learns "Worm! Ugh!" and the next time reacts the same way. A young child may see a grandparent's house burn down and develop an intense fear of fire, even of a lighted match.

The event causing the psychological condition may not be related in any way to the actual problem. For instance, a teenager's parent may die unexpectedly while the young person is attending a school basketball game and he or she may develop a dislike for the sport.

Many psychological problems are manifested by sexual symptoms. If a young man, for example, has an automobile accident following his first intercourse, he might become impotent. Remember that the middle-aged female smoker we talked about earlier was a lonely child who felt accepted by her peers when she smoked that first cigarette on the front lawn. By the time she came to my office, she no longer needed acceptance by a group of young people, but she still smoked.

Bryan defined three clearly recognizable developmental stages of habits or emotional problems:[3]

1. The initial sensitizing event (ISE). The initial sensitizing event may be a conditioning process or a single traumatic occurrence that happens to a person and is forgotten. The ISE usually occurs at a young age, is not recallable by the conscious mind, and produces no symptoms, but it can act as a basis for what will later manifest itself as the problem.

The first time a particular food is eaten, an individual may simply find the taste, the texture, or something about the food unpleasant, but experience no physical reaction. Tomatoes, for example, are a food to which many people are "allergic." The taste of a tomato is unique. It is not a food that would be readily eaten by a child. The first time a small child—let's say a boy—is fed a bite of tomato, he might spit it out.

Although the ISE is not recallable later, the child subconsciously recognizes that he does not like tomatoes. He may, in fact, transfer the dislike to any red, juicy fruit.

Some psychological injuries remain hidden from the conscious mind, and often no symptoms appear. But the subconscious stores up psychological antibodies, and when the subconscious perceives a repetition of the injury, these antibodies pounce (so to speak).

2. The symptom-producing event (SPE). The symptom-producing event can trigger either an emotional or physical reaction, and the individual usually remembers the event. The psychological antigen reacts to the psychological antibodies that were built up by the ISE.

In our example, let's say that a subsequent eating of tomatoes occurs concurrently with another unpleasant experience. Several children are playing near some tomato plants and they see the attractive fruit. They decide to pick and taste one. The event deteriorates into a "hey-these-would-make-good-grenades" behavior in which the youngsters strip the plants of the tomatoes and have a mock battle. The child whose parents were custodians of the tomatoes is punished for being the ringleader in the destructive behavior, and they all are sent to wash up. When the little fellow (whose grandfather had established the tomato plants), washes away the smelly tomato residue, he discovers a rash and runs to his mother for sympathy. The angry parent comments, "It's the acid in those tomatoes. That'll teach you to destroy Grandpop's garden!"

3. The symptom-intensifying event (SIE). When the child attends a community social three years later and his mother hands him a plate and tells him to eat every bite if he wants dessert, he finds himself facing a slice of that offending fruit. He holds his breath and swallows the tomato. And he breaks out in a rash all over. The doctor checks him for various childhood diseases and says lay off the tomatoes. He's happy. He hates tomatoes anyway.

The truth may be that the individual is not physically allergic to tomatoes. His reaction is psychosomatic. Tomatoes are subconsciously connected to that tanning he got in front of his friends at age six.

Symptom-intensifying events are always recallable and such an event may, in fact, be the one that motivates the visit to the doctor or the hypnoanalyst.

Needless to say, I don't see many patients who are worried because they get a rash when they eat tomatoes, but I do see patients whose conditions are caused by a similar progression of events. Hypnoanalysts are faced with solving such questions as: "Why do I have this unreasonable fear of open spaces? I know they are harmless." "Why do I get nauseated every time I go to a basketball game?" "I love my wife; why am I impotent?" "Why can't I get rid of this smoking habit?" "Why do I masturbate everytime I see a pretty girl?"

As a psychotherapist, I was trained in reductionistic techniques designed to help clarify patients' awareness of their problems and, with some patients, alleviate their symptoms. That approach makes for an expensive, drawn-out treatment, and while the patient continues to get symptomatic relief, he or she may still carry around the problem he or she came to me with. Bryan described the hypnoanalytic process as "removing the voltage"[4] of the incident by letting the patient relive it. Once that is cleared up, the patient is usually well. The Bryan hypnoanalytic method is a rapid voltage regulator.

The following multifaceted case is a good example of the order of importance of things in our lives, and the effect of what appeared to be an event unrelated to the presenting symptoms.

He Had a Strange Combination of Symptoms

Dom, a 34-year-old engineering manager, came to my office complaining of several problems: absent-mindedness, difficulty remembering things, inability to spell correctly, being easily distracted on the job, and procrastinating.

I asked how long the problems had existed, and he said, "I've always had them, it's just gotten worse in the last two or three years. I've even been to a neurologist about it since it started getting worse."

I asked what makes it worse, and he said, "I can't say that I can think of anything."

When I asked what makes it better, he said, "Nothing."

I inquired what he had done to help himself, and he repeated that he went to a neurologist who performed a CAT scan and blood tests that turned out negative.

"What do you think you could do after you're cured that you can't do now?" I asked him.

"I think I could be a much-improved contributor to my job and my life, a more effective manager."

Dom did not say that he was having any specific trouble, either with coworkers or with his job. However, when he said that he could be an improved contributor to his job and his life and a more effective manager, he was telling me something: He was experiencing a lack of motivation and was unable to get ahead on the job.

I asked him what traumas had occurred in his life. He recounted that his father had died in the early 1970s, and that he had had a few car accidents. He seemed to put special emphasis on an accident at work four years earlier.

I asked what he wanted from me. He said he wanted to be able to spell words with confidence, routinely remember things, be better organized, and read with improved comprehension.

Now, this was a man who was already fairly successful. He had come to me primarily to improve his memory. He did mention that he had not had a very tough life.

This is the way I summarized his initial sensitizing, symptom-producing, and symptom-intensifying events:

1. His father's death came when he was still a teenager. The event was significant, leaving him without the kind of support and nurturing he needed to become an adult. His father's death, therefore, was a symptom-producing event.

2. He had gotten married and his first boss had died at about the time of his accident at work four years earlier. Those were symptom-intensifying events.

I still had not identified the ISE, so I implemented a word-association test.

Ryan: Fear . . .
Dom: Success.
Ryan: Success . . .
Dom: Remembering.

There evidently was a fear of success and a fear of remembering. Then this question came to mind: "What might he be afraid of remembering?" That was something we needed to determine, so I took this approach:

Ryan: It all started when . . .
Dom: I couldn't remember.
Ryan: It got worse when . . .
Dom: I tried harder.
Ryan: I'm just like . . .

DOM: My dad.

Since his dad was dead, that could have meant that he was feeling dead in some way. Indeed, a part of his mind was dead. He had said that the one thing he needed most was to be able to remember. So we could conclude that, for him, remembering equaled both fear and success. The one thing he needed most? Success.

RYAN: Complete a sentence with the word "why."
DOM: Why can't I relax?
RYAN: I'm afraid when . . .
DOM: I don't remember.
RYAN: Sometimes, I feel like I am stuck at age . . .
DOM: 20.

The major event that affected his life was his father's death when he was 19. He couldn't get beyond age 20.

I returned to the area of guilt in the word associations.

RYAN: Guilt . . .
DOM: Not being able to spell.
RYAN: Punishment . . .
DOM: Not being able to remember.
RYAN: My punishment is . . .
DOM: Not being able to remember.

The major issue here was a death suggestion. A part of the client's mind was killed off when his father died. A secondary problem was the Ponce de Leon syndrome, which we mentioned in Chapter Three. He was stuck being younger than his age. I verified that condition with more word associations:

RYAN: When fire breaks out . . .
DOM: Run.

That is more like what a little kid would say. Most adults don't run when fires break out.

RYAN: Come . . .
DOM: Go.
RYAN: Screw . . .

DOM: Nut.
RYAN: Peter . . .
DOM: Pan.
RYAN: Prick . . .
DOM: Pee pee.

These words with sexual connotations are used because they can help diagnose a Ponce de Leon syndrome. Persons with delayed emotional maturity will make childlike responses.

It was evident that we had several unrelated symptoms to work on. We began working in a subsequent session on his tendency to criticize himself for not remembering or behaving as he thought he should. The criticism problem was fairly easy to deal with under hypnosis. He understood the significance of the behavior and agreed to stop self-criticism.

In a further session, I regressed him to the symptom-producing event, his father's death when Dom was 19 years old. His problem was that his mind had stopped developing at that time. We wiped out the negative experience and brought back to life parts of him that had died with his dad. I coached him and taught him to be his own father, now that he was an adult. He needed to learn to give himself the things he needed. During several sessions we worked rather unsuccessfully on his self-criticism, bad memory, and failure to allow himself to be better.

We did another regression—this time back to when he was in school participating in a type of spelling bee with letters and numbers on the blackboard. He described a situation in which he was embarrassed because he couldn't spell and felt very inadequate. At that time, he apparently had decided that he was not going to spell. We turned that around. He made a decision that he could and would spell correctly. The weak spelling behavior was founded on some erroneous information picked up when he was young, and he decided that he did not want to continue living his life based on something that happened when he was nine years old.

When the patient came to a subsequent session and I asked him how he was doing, he said, "Okay, good. Pretty confident. Still disappointed. I didn't get the promotion."

He had been looking for a promotion.

"He was my mentor and champion," he continued. "He's been out since April. I'm sad and mad. He was a replacement for my father."

Suddenly, we had a broader scenario. Through further questions, I learned that the client's boss had just died and Dom was feeling really bad about it. You may recall that he was still dealing with his father's death, which had occurred more than 10 years earlier, and now he had lost another father figure. This was a real blow to him. We worked on his grief and the loss of the mentor. He continued bringing up the death of his father. Finally, he did agree to be his own father and not look to other people for fathering. He pledged to give himself the love and caring and direction he needed. As we worked out those problems he said he was doing better, that his memory was better, but he still needed to work on his self-confidence and his ability to speak up.

We went back to the spelling bee. As a fourth grader, he had been unable to spell the word "available" and was one of the first to sit down. He drew a significant correlation between his feelings during that spelling bee and being asked in his current business environment to stand up and give presentations.

After we identified and expelled that problem, he began steady improvement. Soon he was actually giving and enjoying presentations before groups. His memory improved and he stopped procrastinating. He was promoted several times during the course of his treatment. He even had his salary increased by 100 percent. He went on to replace the boss who died.

The memory problem was merely a symptom relating to the underlying problem of the need for a father. The initial sensitizing event was the spelling bee. His father's death was the first symptom-producing event; the other events were symptom-intensifying events.

Let's interpret the case: **Dom was willing to give up, to sacrifice something of lesser importance to maintain something of more importance.** He sacrificed his memory skills in order to maintain feelings of love and connectedness to people from the past. The real issue, the underlying diagnosis, had to do with his feelings of love for himself, his feelings of love for his father, and the way that died off when his father died and again when Dom's boss died while he was in treatment.

An interesting sidelight about this case is that his boss was sick and out of work before my patient even came to me for treatment. He did not tell me that until the boss died. That is when the picture finally became clear. His boss's illness and impending death constituted the symptom-intensifying event that caused Dom to come for therapy.

This case was fairly involved, with several concurrent issues stimulating his subconscious mind. I enjoyed working with Dom, who has become very successful since allowing himself to grow up.

WHEN NOTHING ELSE WORKS

Advances have been well documented in treatment of psychoneurotic and psychosomatic conditions through hypnoanalysis. Dr. Bryan claims to have treated 20,000 cases.[5] Hypnoanalysis appears to be solving problems when no other approach has been successful. The roots of depression, anxiety, psychosomatic problems, and phobias can be uncovered through careful hypnoanalytic procedures—history taking, word-association tests, dream analysis, and age regression.

Hypnoanalysis practitioners are not miracle workers. When we ignore the sensationalism from the early days in the field of hypnosis, however, and look at the progress being made today (when the practice is used therapeutically), the conclusion becomes evident: Hypnoanalysis is an important and useful vehicle in health care.

Past-life regression can carry the process one step further. For example: A man with a colon condition worked for years on the psychological and emotional components of his problem as well as the medical aspects—with no success. After being regressed to a life in which he was stabbed to death in the exact spot where the colon was inflamed, he released the feelings connected to that killing and his irritated bowel cleared up.

It seems that this man carried the results of this previous life trauma into his current life. Sound incredible? Yes, but there are numerous case histories of an even more dramatic nature.

Garrett Oppenheim, Ph.D., recounted for the magazine *Contemporary Sexuality* the case of a woman who was having major sexual problems in her relationship with her husband. Under hypnosis, her subconscious produced a memory from a previous life. The woman remembered being a farm girl in the seventeenth century. One day, as she was feeding the pigs, four strangers beat her, raped her, and pushed her into the muck and mud of the pig sty, where she was left to die. Once that memory was exposed to her conscious mind, she was able to overcome her sexual problems with her husband.

Dr. Bryan has recounted a number of fascinating case studies involving past-life regressions. One involved a 33-year-old Australian man who had been impotent all his life. He was treated by a Ukrainian-born hypnotist who had immigrated to Australia, who knew little about the United States, and who spoke English with difficulty.[6]

Under hypnosis, the patient remembered being with General Custer at the Battle of the Little Big Horn. Although this uneducated Australian knew little or nothing about American history, he described the battle and told how he had hidden in a hollow log to escape death. He regarded this as an act of cowardice and carried the guilt with him to his grave. After his death, he remembered, his spirit crossed the Pacific trying to escape the scene of his cowardice. He told of being reborn as an Australian.

His account of the historical event was startlingly accurate in some respects, erroneous in other respects. Dr. Bryan said the historical inaccuracies are no greater than one would expect from someone retelling an event from conscious memory.

Once the Australian had been assured that his act was not born of cowardice but rather from good sense, his subconscious stopped "punishing" him, and his impotence went away.

One of Dr. Bryan's most poignant accounts involved a 22-year-old woman who had once been a bright college student. She sought help after her grades dropped precipitously and her energy and motivation were drowned in a sea of melancholia. Dr. Bryan recognized the walking-zombie syndrome: Something had happened to make her believe she had actually died. Having accepted the death suggestion, she was living out her life as if actually dead.[7]

The symptoms seemed to bear some relation in time to a visit to the dentist. The Muzak system in the dentist's office was playing "The Merry Widow Waltz" as she was administered the gas anesthesia. She felt that if she could be put under gas again she might remember what caused her horror.

She was put into hypnosis and was administered trilene gas as an anesthetic. At first, she associated the awful incident with a concrete ceiling and a room from which she could not exit. After repeated efforts to discover the initial sensitizing event, the horrible episode came to light during a past-life regression: Her subconscious remembered when she was a 14-year-old Jewish girl in Germany. She was sent to Auschwitz, and as she arrived at the train station, a band was playing "The Merry Widow Waltz." She was directed into a room with a concrete ceiling. She was there with many other Jewish prisoners. They thought they were there for a shower. Then, from the shower heads came the gas. Her subconscious remembered the horror of dying in the infamous gas chamber.

Once the memory was expunged from her subconscious the woman—an Irish Catholic born in 1950—was able to return to college and become a good student once more. Dr. Bryan reserved judgment, as I do, on the reality of the past-life experience. But there was no question the woman remembered it as a reality, and by treating it as a reality, he was able to help the patient overcome her problems.

I once had a male patient who always felt a strong aversion toward rape. It was an aversion he told me about only after he had regressed spontaneously to a previous life. He remembered being a woman in India who was raped repeatedly by her husband's relatives on their wedding night. During the regression, he cried and looked quite upset. Afterward, he told me he couldn't understand how any man could force himself on a woman. He said he didn't believe he had it in him, and now he understood why.

IT'S THE FEELINGS THAT COUNT

People act on their emotions, not on their intellect. Hypnoanalysts work to reveal the emotion behind a habit or a behavior. They find the initial sensitizing event (the negative suggestion) in the subconscious mind and take the energy out of it. If a person is depressed, overweight, smoking—whatever the problem is—it means that somewhere in the subconscious mind, a negative suggestion has been accepted. This negative suggestion then is associated with survival, and the patient engages in harmful behavior, thoughts, or feelings to avoid the pain of losing something more important.

In Dom's case, the negative suggestion was that he died when his father died. He felt that he was not grown up and that he couldn't perform as well as his peers. That was true in fourth grade, when he could not spell the word "available," and it was true as an engineering manager who could not remember important things, could not handle the routine expected of him, and could not stand up and give presentations.

Bringing to consciousness the initial sensitizing event neutralized the emotional trigger. It relieved the patient's anxiety and helped him realize he did not need approval and support from his father or a substitute.

Understanding the reason behind a habit is not always necessary in order to deal with it, however. As we will discuss later, depending on the strength of unwanted habits, they can sometimes be changed through self-hypnosis. It's the inflexible ones that must be treated by a specialist.

Key Concepts

- Habits are learned behavior. We establish them by repeated action, but they can be broken.
- Good habits and bad habits are the products of mental conditioning, the result of our subconscious minds having accepted either positive or negative suggestions.
- To be cured of an inflexible, unwanted habit, an individual must relive the emotional incident that caused the problem, reject the negative input lodged there, and accept positive suggestions to replace it.
- The path most of us take in developing our character passes three mileposts: attitudes (beliefs and values) that lead to actions, actions that lead to habits, and habits that lead to life-styles.
- Our attitudes dictate our actions. Through communication from our conscious to our subconscious minds, our actions dictate our habits. And through communication from our subconscious to our conscious minds, our habits dictate our life-styles.
- People are born with only two fears: the fear of falling and the fear of loud noises. All other fears are learned.
- William Jennings Bryan, Jr., M.D., the father of medical hypnoanalysis, defines three clearly recognizable developmental stages of habits or emotional problems: the initial sensitizing event, the symptom-producing event, and the symptom-intensifying event.
- In hypnoanalysis and age regression, we leave all the positive input alone and seek out only the incidents that caused the problem.
- People act on their emotions, not on their intellects. Hypnoanalysts work to reveal the emotion behind a habit or a behavior.
- Bringing to consciousness the initial sensitizing event disarms the emotional trigger.

Growth Exercise

1. List three habits you want to change that are related to the problem(s) that you listed in the exercise at the end of Chapter Three. ___________

____

____

____

2. Make a list of three new habits you'd like to have in your life. _______

____

____

____

3. List the attitudes and actions in your habits that contribute to negativity in your life-style. ______________________________

____

____

____

4. Identify where each habit from question 3 fits into the order of importance listed below.

____

____

   a. Spiritual survival
   b. Psychological survival
   c. Physical survival/air, water, food
   d. Territorial survival
   e. Sexual survival

5. Note what you are sacrificing to maintain something more important.

____

CHAPTER FIVE

STRESS: WHEN REALITY RIOTS

Any man can be
just about as happy
as he makes up his mind
to be.

—*Abraham Lincoln*

WHAT IS STRESS?

Over the last few years, you've probably heard many theories about how stress adversely affects health and well-being. Let's examine exactly what stress is, its warning signs, and how we can cope with it.

Stress is "the nonspecific response of the body to any demand placed upon it."[1] Said another way, stress is a demand upon an organism for change. The change can be perceived as negative or positive. Change is stressful, and since our lives are a succession of changes, stress will always be with us.

Not all stress is negative. Some stress is good. It keeps us alert, interested in life, and motivated to grow. In fact, without stress, we might get little accomplished. The minor emergencies of daily life place demands on our bodies for action. Reacting positively to these situations is stressful but manageable. Thus, normal stress provides the stimuli that keeps us going in everyday living.

Our bodies were designed to deal with stress in a fight-or-flight mode. When our ancestors saw a bear or a lion, they had to make up their minds whether to fight or run for their lives. In either case, their bodies needed an extra charge of energy to get them through the emergency. They also needed a mechanism to turn off the extra energy when the threat had passed. Our bodies are still designed to provide that extra voltage when challenges are perceived. But the challenge rarely comes in the form of a physical threat that requires us either to fight or to run. The "threat" may be the mail carrier arriving with a handful of bills or an audit notice from the Internal Revenue. In such cases, we feel the stress, but neither fighting nor fleeing will remove the threat. So we find ourselves in situations in which we're energized for action but have no means of discharging the extra energy. When this happens, we experience "distress," caused by the excessive accumulation of pent-up emotional and physical responses.

There Are Limits

Our ability to cope with stress changes from time to time throughout life. Depending largely on the type, amount, duration, and intensity of stress each of us experiences, we may reach a critical limit, a personal point that differs for each individual.

As an example: Leah's parents were concerned over her behavioral problems and her astral projection powers—the ability to separate her spiritual and physical beings and leave her body at will. The 15-year-old girl described family relations with typical teenage frustration and anger. Her conversation was splattered with four-letter words, posturing, and impulsive statements. She indicated her chief problem was not her out-of-body experiences, but that her parents blamed her for her sister's problems, that they had turned her into a go-between—a "telephone operator," she called it.

The parental pressure had started three years earlier, Leah said, when her sister began dating a boy they disapproved of. Leah tried to solve the conflict by discussing the matter with them and altering her own behavior so as to worry them even more. She said:

> I talked to them and stopped bringing home nice boys and tried bringing home some assholes. And I want to kill them. . . . It stops me from going out with nice guys, and I won't go out with anybody.

In other words, she was sacrificing herself, sacrificing her dating life to maintain stability in her family—something more important to her.

Two facets of this case were particularly interesting. I asked Leah to describe herself, and she said she was a brat. "I don't really get into it. I just do it to do it," she said.

She also said she was born with cranial stenosis (the absence of the normal soft spot in her head). She had two operations for the condition, first at 6 months, and again at 18 months.

Then she revealed the clincher, again with typical teenage lack of focus. I asked what she wanted from me and she said:

> I want to find out what my past lives were. A lot of things freak me out. I have this power. I came up like a light and turned into 5,000 lights. I want to learn to control it. I want to lose weight and I want to get better in school so they [her parents] quit coming down on me.

How's that for an assignment?

Leah went on to talk about her out-of-body experiences, saying that her spirit leaves her body many, many times at night and travels around. I knew I could do nothing about her parents "coming down on her," as she called it, but I could help her learn to deal with the astral projections and to stop sacrificing herself to maintain the family telephone-operator position.

I regressed her to the first time she left her body. She was in the hospital at six or seven months and recovering from surgery to her head. This is what she said:

> It hurts across the top of my head. It's painful. I am thinking, "Why is this happening?" I am waking up from it. It hurts a lot.

We discussed the fact that her headaches were a kind of subconscious proof that she was alive and that her out-of-body experiences originally were attempts to escape physical pain and continued as a way of escaping emotional pain. Under hypnosis, we removed the pain she had felt and helped her to understand that she no longer had to be the family go-between.

Actually, Leah ended up being mad at me. By understanding the unconscious reasons for which she was practicing astral projection, she lost the ability to leave her body. She had only wanted to control it.

Leah is doing very well 18 months after treatment. She has changed schools, is making good grades, and is dating appropriate types of persons. "I've got the little kid out of me," she said.

Even though Leah was curious about her previous lives, I did not take her through a past-life regression, simply because it wasn't necessary to complete the treatment. I will regress a person to past lives only if the treatment warrants it or if the patient requests it after the initial problems have been solved. Most problems can be resolved without past-life regressions. It's important that the hypnoanalyst know when and how to initiate the regression.

STRESS MANIFESTS ITSELF IN MANY WAYS

Many conditions that we call diseases are actually psychosomatic illnesses caused by stress. Psychosomatic illness results when a part of the body fails to function properly—not because of infection or disease, but because of tension or distress. When stress has reached the saturation point, you send a signal to yourself warning you to slow down. Those signals include tension, sore muscles, irritability, backache, fatigue, depression, listlessness, disinterest in what is happening around you, overeating, drinking too much, heart palpitations, or digestive problems such as cramps, gas, and diarrhea. You may fail to recognize those stress signals until a crisis confronts you, forcing you to admit to and possibly deal with an overstressed condition.

There are situations in life with a high stress value that you may not even be aware of. T. H. Holmes and R. H. Rahe developed a stress-evaluation test called the "Social Readjustment Rating Scale," which lists many possibilities for stress and appoints a life-change units (LCU) number value to each.[2] The Holmes-Rahe scale is a good tool for predicting distress. For example, on the top of the list is the death of a spouse (100 points). The last item is a minor violation of the law (11 points), with everything from pregnancy, change in financial state, loss of job, and change in sleeping habits to the beginning and ending of school in between.

The idea is to total the LCU point values of the stressors in your life. A score of 300 or more means an 80 percent chance of illness. Any time you score more than 150 on the test, you are probably experiencing distress that could result in an associated health change. The test can be used to develop your "Stress Quotient." Everyone is unique and will have different quotients. Figure out what yours is, and when you find yourself approaching that level, take action to reduce the stress you are experiencing. Let's look at the Holmes-Rahe scale in its entirety (see Figure 5.1).

Medical research has shown that stress is a major factor in about 75 percent of all illnesses. Knowing how much pressure and tension you can cope with and when and how to reduce it will help you avoid health-threatening or even life-threatening situations. The correlation between stress and heart disease has caused many heart specialists to recommend relaxation therapy to patients at high risk for coronary problems. The severe stress that follows the death of a spouse leaves the survivor more than twice as vulnerable to illness or accidents as the average person. The following case illustrates that type of situation.

Stress Plays Major Role

James and Lucille had been married more than 50 years and had reared six children when she developed a heart problem. Bypass surgery was performed, and she returned to her home. He nursed her.

Then she had a stroke. She spent several weeks in a hospital and therapy center before returning to the house in a wheelchair. He nursed her, assisted by a housekeeper through the week and daughters who traveled more than 100 miles to help out on weekends.

When Lucille died, James was at loose ends. He played lots of golf, attended to business investments, and visited his children. One of his daughters was a single professional with more than 20 years at her position. He tried to talk her into giving up her job and moving back home to live with him. When she refused, he married Estelle.

Estelle's husband had died about a month after Lucille's death. The two couples had known each other in church and community functions. James and Estelle both needed companionship. It seemed like a good idea. She rented out her house, and they planned to live in his and Lucille's home.

Social Readjustment Rating Scale

Rank	Life event	Mean value
1	Death of a spouse	100
2	Divorce	73
3	Marital separation	65
4	Jail term	63
5	Death of a close family member	63
6	Personal injury or illness	53
7	Marriage	50
8	Fired at work	47
9	Marital reconciliation	45
10	Retirement	45
11	Change in health of family member	44
12	Pregnancy	40
13	Sex difficulties	39
14	Gain of new family member	39
15	Business readjustment	39
16	Change in financial state	38
17	Death of close friend	37
18	Change to different line of work	36
19	Change in number of arguments with spouse	35
20	Mortgage over $10,000	31
21	Foreclosure of mortgage or loan	30
22	Change in responsibilities at work	29
23	Son or daughter leaving home	29
24	Trouble with in-laws	29
25	Outstanding personal achievement	28
26	Wife begins or stops work	26
27	Begin or end school	26
28	Change in living conditions	25
29	Revision of personal habits	24
30	Trouble with boss	23
31	Change in work hours or conditions	20
32	Change in residence	20
33	Change in schools	20
34	Change in recreation	19
35	Change in church activities	19
36	Change in social activities	18
37	Mortgage or lien less than $10,000	17
38	Change in sleeping habits	16
39	Change in number of family get-togethers	15
40	Change in eating habits	15
41	Vacation	13
42	Christmas	12
43	Minor violations of the law	11

Figure 5.1

Upon returning from their honeymoon, Estelle opened a door in James's unfamiliar house and tumbled down a set of stairs. She received multiple fractures of a wrist and several bad bruises and was confined to bed for a few weeks. James nursed her.

Shortly after Estelle was up on her feet again, James suffered a mild heart attack. "Nothing serious," the doctor said. "He'll be up and about soon." In the meantime, he had to miss the annual Labor Day family reunion held by Lucille's family, an event he had always enjoyed and his one opportunity to visit with long-time in-laws.

"That was probably best," he said. "Lucille's sisters might resent Estelle's presence and I would hate to leave her alone for the day."

Three months later, he experienced a massive heart attack and died.

"He's had a hard time of it," his children said.

Add up James's life-change unit score. He was piling change on top of change. Is it any wonder he succumbed?

WHAT CAN WE DO ABOUT IT?

All right, now that we know what stress is and what its symptoms are, how do we cope? We can avoid stress in many ways. The easiest route to controlling minor stress is to talk to someone. Sharing problems and ways of coping starts you off on the road to success. You will benefit more than you might think by understanding how others are coping.

Hypnosis is another safe method of stress reduction. It does not utilize drugs and is often the quickest way to teach people to relax and manage their stress. In addition to seeking out a sympathetic listener or utilizing hypnosis, other ways to cope with stress include:

- Avoiding too many changes at once, especially those with high LCUs.
- Thinking of options (break routines by using your creative problem-solving ability).
- Scheduling fun times into your normal activities.
- Taking up some aerobic activity (dancing, walking, running, swimming).

- Utilizing hypnosis tapes. There are several good tapes on the market. I have one called "Relax the Worry and Tension Away." Or you can make your own, as we will discuss later.
- Practicing deep-breathing exercises combined with visual imagery or yoga.
- Listening to baroque music (Vivaldi, Correlli, and others). It has a 60-cycle beat, which is calming.
- Soaking in a hot tub or using a sauna.
- Following a proper diet—avoiding junk foods and sugar.
- Getting your mind off yourself by doing something for others.
- Practicing meditation or prayer.
- Getting involved in nonverbal expression through art, clay, dance, mime.
- Setting priorities.
- Learning flexibility and avoiding rigidity.
- Taking regular naps.
- Giving up trying to be perfect.
- Escaping through books, movies, or plays.
- Getting or giving massages, sharing nurturing and hugs.

The power of the hug should not be underestimated. It is one of the most potent methods for healing emotional wounds, relieving stress, and building self-esteem.

The person who receives an abundance of warm hugs during childhood grows up with more confidence and poise, more self-esteem, and greater ability to cope with life's challenges. The person starved for hugs grows up with a constant need for outside stimulation to keep morale and self-esteem up.

The hug is a powerful generator of beta endorphins, those substances, manufactured in various parts of the body, that have a soothing effect on certain receptors in the brain. Endorphins are also produced by strenuous exercise and are the source of the "jogger's high."

Greg Risberg, M.S.W., a therapist, consultant and speaker, is an authority on hugs. He identified seven types of hugs at a seminar he gave and which I attended.[3]

The first is the A-frame hug. In this type of hug, the shoulders of the hugger and the huggee barely touch. Trying to activate the beta endorphin pump through this type of hug is like trying to activate your automobile's starter when there's a bad battery connection.

The one-side hug is little better. In this type of clinch, the two partners touch closely at one shoulder, but the hugger is still held at a distance.

The two-sided hug is a little better. Both shoulders touch, but the lower torsos are still apart.

The shoulder-to-waist hug begins to establish a better connection. In this clinch, the partners stand closer, and the huggee no longer holds the hugger away, though their lower trunks still don't touch.

Next comes the shoulder-to-pelvis hug, and we're starting to get there. The endorphins are flowing freely, and before they're aware of it, the partners may be into the shoulder-to-knees hug. The observer can barely distinguish this one from the biggest endorphin-pumper of them all—the shoulder-to-the-tips-of-the-toes-and-everywhere-in-between hug. Do it with someone you love, or who needs your love, and see if you both don't feel a lot better for it.

STRESS FROM LONG AGO

In my work as a hypnoanalyst, I treat people all the time who are suffering from stress and anxiety. Though not all of my clients are adults, most are. Yet, I often discover that the event that triggered their current stress occurred in childhood, sometimes in infancy, at birth, or even in intrauterine life.

STRESS HAS MULTIPLE EFFECTS

In his newsletter, Dr. Louis K. Boswell reports that researchers at the University of Wisconsin have documented reduced immune responses (lasting for several weeks) in baby monkeys that were separated from their mothers. When they were isolated, the young primates experienced altered white blood cell counts, making them more susceptible to illness. "Study of this particular stress response in monkeys has revealed the probability of long-term effects of early-life stress," Boswell concludes. "Infant isolation due to divorce, hospitalization, or the death or prolonged absence of either parent could yield unhealthy consequences in later life."[4]

Diane's Symptom Was Fatigue

Diane, an attorney by profession, came to me complaining of chronic fatigue, lack of motivation, and difficulty getting up in the morning. A young mother, she had not worked outside the home for four or five years, which corresponded to the duration of the fatigue and other symptoms. She procrastinated, she said, about the things she should be doing in favor of creative activities she enjoyed.

According to Diane, her life was about perfect. She had everything she had wanted and worked for. She loved her husband and her children, was happy with her religion, and had a perfect house in a perfect community. She just didn't know why she was so tired and had no motivation, why she couldn't structure a fulfilling day for herself when everything around her was so great.

Diane's history told of a number of troubling experiences. A bout with cancer had resulted in mastectomies. When she was a girl living at home, her sister had suffered a mental breakdown. Her mother had died when Diane was 26, and her brother had died when she was 30.

I asked whether there were any problems when her mother was carrying her. She told me that right after she was born, her mother had had a mastectomy and a hysterectomy. For three to six weeks during that family crisis, the infant Diane had been cared for in the home of her aunt Maye.

Her feelings of guilt, she told me, were associated with the things she didn't do. Her expectation from hypnoanalysis was that she would feel more energy and would stop procrastinating.

I age regressed Diane and learned that her birth trauma and her separation from her mother were the initial sensitizing events (ISEs) out of which her current problem had grown. The deaths of her mother and brother and her mastectomies were symptom-producing events. Giving birth to her children and giving up her professional life-style to stay home were symptom-intensifying events.

As is often the case, Diane's symptoms were due to both physical and emotional disorders contributing to each other. She had chosen a "flight" response to her situation. The fight-or-flight response, you will recall, is a built-in survival mechanism that helps you defend yourself or escape from threatening situations. If you do not constructively deal with the challenge, it will deal with you destructively. This is what had happened with Diane.

Although she had freely decided on motherhood over career, her self-esteem was suffering and she responded by neglecting creative activities in favor of doing everyday household chores.

Diane's symptoms, after first disappearing, eventually reappeared. At her request, I did a past-life regression, which helped us find out what retriggered them.

Here are the young attorney's responses to her treatment and her description of the hypnoanalytic process:

> At the time I came in for treatment, I felt [my fatigue and low motivation] was at 10 on a 1-10 scale. . . . I didn't understand why I couldn't handle it. For about a month after treatment, I didn't feel the problem existed at all, then I noticed it creeping in a little [2 on a scale of 10]. I felt [the resurgence] had to do with a past life, what I saw, how I died in a war situation. I felt that I carried self-pity into this life, but I think I've worked it out with self-hypnosis.
>
> I found the [hypnosis] process fascinating. Two of the weeks when I learned I had a death wish and negative feelings about women were anxious and difficult. My conscious mind didn't want to believe this about myself. . . . I found all the positive reinforcement was relaxing and peaceful.

The death wish she spoke of was the walking-zombie syndrome.

Asked if she experienced any unusual events, side effects, or circumstances during treatment, Diane said:

> Seeing a past life, pregnancy, labor, and delivery was unusual for me.
>
> Hypnosis has to be the single most important thing I've done for myself in my lifetime.
>
> Though I felt something was holding me back, I didn't think I was crazy or mentally ill, and I didn't think my situation warranted traditional treatment. [Hypnoanalysis] clarified what the problem was and took care of it. Prior to [hypnoanalysis], I had been walking around feeling dead inside, but not realizing it, since this was all I had known.
>
> After hypnoanalysis, I feel energetic and alive. It eliminated my feelings of self-doubt and I became more creative. Good things started happening to me at the same time. Once, I had a dream and its theme was that I was afraid to live and afraid to die. I'm not afraid of either anymore. Life is more fulfilling now, and I'm sure death will be also.

Age regression under hypnosis can help both patient and therapist define events that contribute to psychosomatic disorders, such as Diane's extreme fatigue, occurring in adulthood. Because these symptoms are so often present among the young professional population, this particular syndrome is often referred to as the "yuppy" disease.

POSTTRAUMATIC STRESS DISORDER IS COMMON

Another familiar manifestation of psychosomatic illness is Posttraumatic Stress Disorder (PTSD). PTSD has been around under different names for generations. It is most often suffered by victims and witnesses of such disasters as hurricanes and earthquakes, criminal assault, accidents, war, and other violence. Following World War II, for example, we said returning vets were suffering from "shell shock." Work with Vietnam veterans produced the PTSD appellation. More recently, people who claim to have been abducted by aliens also tend to exhibit similar responses.

Sean Blamed Himself for His Buddy's Death

Sean, 40, entered my office in a wheelchair. He had lost his legs in Vietnam. When I asked what the problem was, he said:

> Two things. About two weeks ago, I really flew off the handle. I grabbed my wife and son.

Then he added:

> I just wanted to get to the bottom of it. Things I had let build up and didn't tell anybody about.

He hesitated, then went on:

> Intense rage. I had headaches for about 10 years. The last two days I haven't had them. I've felt more relaxed ever since I started smoking.

I asked how long his temper had been a problem, and he said in an emotional voice:

> It wasn't temper—rage. It was real different. It just came up. Boom. A combination of things that just built.

He said that nothing made it worse, but cigarettes made it better. When I asked what he had done to help himself, he responded:

> Looking inward. Putting myself back on track. Meditation.

I asked what he thought he would be able to do once he was cured that he could not do now, and he thoughtfully replied: "Not always be putting myself out on a limb and carrying the rest of the world's problems." He paused, then added: "I want to find the cause [for the rage] and then I will know for sure that it will not happen again." Another pause.

"It doesn't bother me any more." He looked toward heaven. "It's 21 years. I was hit in Vietnam in 1966. A fencepost. Two others died. I was the most severely wounded. I heard my buddy screaming, 'God, don't let me die.'"

I found myself unprepared for a war-ravaged 40-year-old paraplegic's response to my query about traumatic events in his life. I had expected the loss of his legs to be the chief issue, but when I asked what hurt him most, he again looked upward and said:

> The divorce was a bummer, a heavy one. The death of my father, a real heavy one. I miss him. When I was 11.

I waited without comment and he picked back up:

> I wouldn't call Vietnam traumatic. I saved a little girl from drowning. That first 12 hours was real rough.

You will recall that his first word to me was "two." He said that two things were problems. The number kept showing up all over the place during the history taking.

I asked him about drugs and he said, "No, I was on morphine every two hours for two weeks when I was in the hospital."

I asked him about eating. He reported that he "tries to eat two meals a day."

Children? "I have two."

He told me he spent 30 months in the hospital after Vietnam, losing 100 pounds. That, he said, was traumatic. He also reported that he was born two months prematurely, nearly drowned when he was 6 or 7 years old, had kidney stones when he was 13, and yellow jaundice at some time. And he commented that his childhood was fantastic.

He could not recall any early memories of his mother, who was in a nursing home at the time he came to me. "She hugged me only once, after my dad's death," he offered, but added that he had been close to his grandparents, who died when he was 12 or 13.

When asked about any guilt feelings, he listed only his friend's death in Vietnam. "I wasn't able to help him," he said.

When I asked what he wanted from me, he said simply, "resolution of why the rage was there."

So, in the word-association test, we were looking for an ISE in Sean's past that caused a lot of rage to develop.

RYAN: The real problem . . .
SEAN: Not being able to relax.
RYAN: One thing I need most is . . .

Sean: To relax.
Ryan: Birth . . . (Note Sean's response.)
Sean: Hanging.
Ryan: What I don't want you to know is . . .
Sean: There are men killed.
Ryan: Because I couldn't help him . . .
Sean: He died.
Ryan: It all started when . . .
Sean: Childhood.

From his responses, it appeared that his birth felt like death and was probably the initial sensitizing event. It also appears that he experiences guilt over having killed in Vietnam.

While he was under hypnosis, I explained my sense of his problem and regressed him back to the womb. Sean's was the most emotional experience I have ever seen while working with a person under hypnosis. Although he was reclined in the chair, he kept rising, screaming, and writhing while reliving the experience.

At six or seven months inside the womb, he said:

> It's warm. I am in breech position. My head under the sternum. Uncomfortable. (He was evidently in pain.)
>
> It must be time for me to be born. My chest hurts. It's hard to breathe. I am stopped in the canal. It's pressure on my lungs. A lot of pain. I'm scared, need help. I'm coming out. I'm out, but I passed out. They're turning me over, cleaning me off. It's cold, it's cold. They're wrapping me up. (Sean starts shaking all over and making a lot of noise.)
>
> They're not getting the ice, the ice off me. They lay me down on my back, Mom's left side. Warm, but hard to catch my breath. I can't see, it's dark and scary.

I had him leave his traumatic feelings from birth in the past, along with any association with them that was connected in his here and now.

In the next session, he reported feeling good, not getting easily upset.

During another visit, I regressed Sean to a time when he was drowning. He recalled:

> We were swimming in a natural reservoir. I slipped through an inner tube. It didn't bother me, though I couldn't breathe. My brother pulled me up, then I got scared. He was coughing up water.

I removed this death suggestion from his subconscious. However, here was the ISE for his feeling of responsibility for other people.

Then, we took care of his case of survivor guilt. I regressed him back to Vietnam and asked him to stop blaming and punishing himself for the deaths of his two friend. At this point, he let go of his spiritual death wish.

Once these situations were reviewed and the effect on the subconscious nullified, Sean was freed up enough to stop treatment. My preference was to give him a few more reinforcements, but, as my mother used to say, "The proof is in the pudding." Two years later, Sean continues to do well and has not reexperienced the rage toward his family that so frightened him.

The number two that kept coming up seemed to refer to the two deaths in Vietnam. Had he continued in treatment, I would have known for sure. Frequently, but not always, numbers that show up repeatedly are significant.

When Sean relived the Vietnam scene, I wept from the pain of hearing it. Here was a man who was nearly blown to pieces himself—a man so gravely injured that he would never again walk on his own legs. Yet his thoughts were on his buddies, and his concern for them haunted his subconscious for years afterward.

SYMPTOMS AND TREATMENT OF PTSD

War veterans are not the only persons experiencing posttraumatic conditioning, of course. The young survivors of Israeli-Palestinian conflicts whom you see on the evening news scurrying amid the rubble are candidates for PTSD, aren't they? How about victims of the Persian Gulf War, the latest earthquake, or the most recent hurricane? The Holmes-Rahe scale provides a long list of other traumatic events that many or all of us will face in our lifetime. While such occurrences as death of a spouse or family member, divorce, or changing jobs are not life threatening and are not considered to cause PTSD, they are, nonetheless, traumatic.

Dr. Boswell lists the following symptoms routinely experienced by PTSD sufferers:[5]

- They persistently reexperience the traumatic event in nightmares and flashbacks and experience marked distress at exposure to symbolic events. They are invaded by thoughts of the past event.
- Because their nervous systems are conditioned to respond to particular stimuli, they are plagued by persistent, increased arousal, making it difficult for them to sleep, concentrate, or control anger. They may also have an exaggerated startle response.

- They avoid any place, person, or thing that would arouse memory of the traumatic event, thus limiting their ability to have a successful career, marriage, or future plans.

I guide patients suffering from PTSD back to the ISE and work with them in recognizing and leaving the trauma there in the past. This opens their minds to dealing with the major traumatic event in their lives. I then offer gentle suggestions to help them reshape their lives. Hypnoanalysis helps PTSD victims cope with present and future problems in a positive, effective manner. If we fail to kick out the problem causing the stress, many PTSD sufferers resort to alcohol, drugs, or other antisocial behavior, which provide short-term relief but translate into more long-term problems.

Key Concepts

- Stress, as defined by Hans Selye, is "the nonspecific response of the body to any demand" placed upon it.
- Not all stress is negative. Without stress, we might get little accomplished. Normal stress is the challenge of everyday living.
- Our bodies were designed to deal with stress in a fight-or-flight mode. When reacting to normal stress appropriately, a charge and discharge mechanism operates and relieves the stress.
- Distress is the excessive accumulation of pent-up emotional and physical responses to routine anxieties and tension or to traumatic events.
- Our ability to cope with stress changes from time to time throughout life. Depending largely on the type, amount, duration and intensity of stress each of us experiences, we may reach a critical limit, a personal point that differs for each individual.
- Psychosomatic illness results when tension or distress interferes with the proper functioning of some part of our bodies.
- Medical research has shown that stress is a major factor in about 75 percent of all illnesses.
- The easiest route to minor stress control is to talk to someone.
- Hypnosis is another safe method of stress reduction.
- Events from childhood, infancy, the period inside the womb, or even from a previous life are factors affecting stress in adulthood.
- The isolation of an infant resulting from divorce or hospitalization, or the death or prolonged absence of either parent, can cause unhealthy consequences in later life.
- Age regression under hypnosis can help both patient and therapist locate events that contribute to psychosomatic disorders.
- Posttraumatic Stress Disorder (PTSD) is often suffered by victims of criminal assault, accidents, war, and other violence, and by witnesses of such natural disasters as hurricanes and earthquakes.

Growth Exercise

1. Take the stress test and note your score. ____________________

2. The following list names many of the symptoms of too much stress. Check off those that apply.

   — Feeling harried, hurrying around; driving, talking, eating faster than usual

   — Feeling bored, apathetic, depressed, listless, no energy

   — Disturbances in sleeping or eating patterns

   — Chronic dissatisfaction

   — Having no fun, lack of interest in sex

   — Perfectionism, perfidiousness, workaholism, etc.

   — Accident proneness

   — Feeling victimized by your life, decisions, etc.

CHAPTER SIX

RELAXATION: TURNPIKE TO THE SUBCONSCIOUS

The empires of the future are the empires of the mind.

—*Winston Churchill*

IT'S REALLY VERY EASY

Sometimes, complicated concepts are actually very simple. That is the case with relaxation and self-hypnosis. You can utilize the process to boost your self-esteem and to program your mind for whatever you want in your life. In my practice, I encourage it for reinforcement and I teach patients to use it for continued growth following hypnoanalysis.

Self-hypnosis will not enable you to perform magic or display talents that you do not already possess; but it will enable you to develop new skills, create life situations, and deal creatively with stress. It will also help you overcome blocks and self-imposed limitations that prevent you from making the best use of your abilities and talents. Hypnosis will help you develop your latent potential.

Self-hypnosis is a natural exercise that most of us practice regularly. We develop habits through self-hypnosis or mental conditioning. Because of past programming, many of us function on automatic pilot more than we realize. If we did something a certain way 10 years ago, it's a safe bet we do it the same way today, unless a crisis has forced us to change, or unless we've decided a change is necessary because of the consequences ahead of us.

Through subconscious mental conditioning, we move through rooms in our house without telling our arms to reach out and our hands to turn the knobs. Our feet hit the brake automatically when we drive into touchy traffic situations. We awake at our preferred time daily.

EASY DOES IT

Relaxation is the key to reprogramming and self-hypnosis, the key that opens the door to taking control of your attitudes, your behavior, and the stress in your life. Relaxation is a normal state. Being tense requires energy. The choice is yours. It does have to be a total body-mind experience, however. You cannot be physically relaxed while mentally tense, or vice versa.

Achieving a relaxed state is a skill that we all knew as babies but that most of us have forgotten by adulthood, so let's explore the process. Simple deep breathing is the easiest road to relaxation. Deep breathing is a natural stress reliever. It counteracts the fight-or-flight response and restores the body to its normal functioning. Typical, shallow breathing actually contributes to a distressed state, while deep breathing helps ward off distress before it begins by keeping the body and mind relaxed.

Let's look at the process of self-hypnosis as a way to program your mind. After you have practiced these simple steps a few times, you will be able to achieve a relaxed state at will:

1. Deep breathing. Most people breathe from their chests rather than from their diaphragms. Your diaphragm separates the chest from the abdomen. Deep breathing is an asset if you want to reprogram your mind and develop a healthy life practice. Shallow breathing cuts down on oxygen intake and encourages muscle tension. Hyperventilation, the opposite of relaxation, results from rapid, shallow breathing. Follow these steps to become adept at deep breathing:

a. Choose a very quiet location, lie down, and get comfortable.

b. Place your hands just below your rib cage and inhale deeply through your nose. Your hands should move up and down rhythmically as you breathe in and breathe out.

c. Exhale, through your mouth, as completely as you inhale. Concentrate on emptying your lungs. Practice inhaling through your nose and exhaling through your mouth until you are comfortable with the pattern.

2. Relaxing. Relaxation is a progressive event throughout the body. While you are in your quiet spot, follow these steps to achieve total body relaxation:

a. Lie down, or sit in a straight-backed chair, and tense your entire body.

b. Relax your body, **one part at a time**, starting with your feet. Concentrate on relaxing your feet, then move up and concentrate on relaxing your ankles, then your calves. Follow the procedure up through your knees, thighs, abdomen, trunk, hands, arms, shoulders, neck, and face, relaxing only one body area at a time.

c. You can condition yourself to go into a deep-breathing, relaxed state by adopting a cue and repeating it as you achieve relaxation. Keep saying over and over "I'm relaxed and calm," or whatever phrase is comfortable for you. "I'm cool and awesome" is acceptable if that will do it. Eventually, you can rapidly achieve a relaxed state by simply using the cue. That's self-hypnosis in action.

3. Imaging. After your body is relaxed, you can relax your mind through daydreaming. Let your thoughts wander to pleasant environs, quiet places, a setting that creates feelings of comfort and tranquility. Maybe it's a favorite spot by a quiet stream; maybe it's in front of a warm fire.

Daydreaming fits right into the suggestive relaxation pattern. It makes you feel good about yourself and conditions your subconscious for reprogramming. When you are completely absorbed in something, you are unaware of time or what is going on around you. Your mind cannot concentrate on two things at once. Thus, if it is focused on a pleasant, positive image, it cannot be preoccupied with negative thoughts. In this state, your subconscious is freed up and receptive to creative activity.

4. Visualizing. Mental programming can take place at this stage. The conscious mind must be in a passive state for the subconscious to accept programming. A focused state of attention (sometimes called a trance) creates the best conditions for accepting self-suggestions. This state is in the alpha level of awareness. You are fully cognizant of what is going on around you, but are concentrating by choice on a matter of importance, and are creating mental images of what you want to happen. Visualize the situation you want. Be sure to use the present tense. If you want to lose weight, "see" a slim you in a smashing new swimsuit, strolling on the beach, being ogled by members of the opposite sex, or at a party being complimented on your appearance. If you want to stop smoking, imagine yourself facing the urge to smoke but overcoming the desire and breathing deeply and freely without coughing. If you want to rid yourself of your fear of water, visualize yourself swimming confidently in cool, clear water, enjoying the refreshing sense one gets from a mountain pool. If you want to overcome illness, visualize yourself strong and healthy, participating in your favorite physical activity.

For more details on the techniques of self-hypnosis, turn to Appendix A in the back of this book.

Remember the old expression, "Seeing is believing"? I think it is the other way around: Believing is seeing. You will see what you believe you are going to see. You bring to a situation what you expect you are going to experience. Visualization activates the subconscious mind. It puts you in charge of your life. The subconscious does not recognize the difference between fantasy and reality. You will be what you visualize that you will be. There's an old saying: "Whatever the mind can conceive and believe, it can achieve."

What you actually see merely validates your belief system. If, as a salesperson, you believe that the winter months are slow months, if you verbalize, "It doesn't make any difference what I do this time of year, people don't buy my product around the Christmas season . . . all the other salespeople have it slow too this time of year," you will subconsciously look for and consciously see only the evidence that your belief is true. You will see numerous indications that business is down during the winter months and likely notice very little that is going right or think of little you can do to increase your business. Thus, your belief is validated and continues to strengthen. It may be that your competitors prefer a slow Christmas season because they like to go duck hunting on the Chesapeake Bay or spend time with their families. Consequently, you create a self-fulfilling prophecy.

Based on the concept that "believing is seeing," you can consciously choose what will show up in your life, regardless of your chosen profession. The game of life is not a game of chance, but a game of choice—and the choice is yours.

DIFFERENT TYPES OF IMAGERY

The use of imagery enables you to "create" memories. Most of us indulge in spontaneous imagination, when we turn our minds loose to roam at will. The daydreams that thus occur are similar to night dreams: We do not plan them or direct them. It's like the involuntary recalling of a memory.

But you can use your conscious mind to create the scenes or the circumstances you would like to exist. This is called "willed imagination." You construct your own daydream, imagining things as you would like them to be. The image thus created becomes fixed in your memory as firmly as if you had actually lived through it. Your subconscious accepts this memory as reality and directs your responses accordingly.

For most people, a daydream is like an image projected on a movie screen. They're observers and not participants in the scene. In his book *Imagineering for Health*, author Serge King calls this "picture imagination." Another form of imagery is what King calls "mime imagination." Through it, you become a participant rather than an observer.[1]

To illustrate: Picture a dashing new sports car parked beneath the palm trees on some sunny beach. Let it be the make and model of your choice. You get into the car. You turn the ignition. The engine roars to life. You snap it into first gear, engage the clutch, give it the gas, and feel the back of the seat pressing against your back as the car accelerates. You've just experienced "picture imagination."

Now step out into your driveway. Picture that same car sitting in front of you. Imagine your real hands opening that door. Imagine yourself sliding into that seat and driving the car down the familiar streets of your neighborhood. You have now brought your image out of never-never land and into your here and now. This is "mime imagination."

As King points out, picture imagination is good for memory recall, for developing new ideas, for planning projects, and for various types of meditation. Mime imagination is best for improving your personality and skills in your relationships, in your environment, and in your health. Athletes use it to prepare themselves for competition through polishing their techniques and instilling self-confidence.

Imagery can involve much more than mental pictures. You can imagine tastes, smells, sounds, and feelings as well.

When you imagine the smell of coffee brewing in the morning, of roses perfuming a country lane, or of salt air and suntan lotion on a sunny beach, you are using olfactory imagery. When you imagine the taste of a banana split, of saltwater taffy, or of a filet mignon topped with bearnaise, you are using gustatory imagery. These forms of imagery can be used to "create" pleasant experiences.

Auditory and kinesthetic imagery are more powerful ways of visualizing the things you want. Auditory imagery involves the sense of hearing. You imagine the sound of surf crashing against a beach, of birds singing in a garden, of rain pattering on the rooftop. Kinesthetic energy involves the sense of touch. You can imagine the coolness of the water as you first dive into a pool, the bracing warmth of a hot shower at the end of a weary day, the feel of the wind and the snow as you ski down a spectacular slope, and the solid feel of bat meeting ball as you swing for the fence.

Individuals vary as to the type of imagery they prefer. The hypnoanalyst's task is to determine which type predominates in a particular patient. The analyst can use this knowledge to communicate more effectively with the patient.

The therapist can determine the patient's preferred mode of imagery by listening carefully to the verbs the patient uses. A person who uses words such as "look," "see," "bright," and "dark" is saying, "I prefer visual imagery." The patient who uses words such as "feel," "heavy," "light," "pressure," "grasp," or "hold," is saying, "I prefer kinesthetic imagery." People who use words such as "hear," "say to myself," "talking," "sounds like," and "tune in" are signaling that they prefer auditory imagery.

The therapist responds by using similar words in communicating with the patient. The patient thus can understand the therapist better and knows, intuitively, that the understanding is mutual.[2]

Keep these tips in mind to boost your visualization effectiveness:

- Repeat your visualizations. Repetition etches the image into your subconscious mind.
- Practice often. Frequent practice leads to improvement. By choosing the same time daily, you can make a habit of self-hypnosis.
- Maintain control over your imagery. Say no to undesired images and feelings.
- Continue to breathe from your diaphragm during your visualization periods to maintain your relaxed state.
- Be sure to create the exact feeling that your goal will produce in you, thereby associating the image with the feeling and keeping in mind that the intensity of the subconscious program depends on your feelings.

If you have trouble with imagination, if you can't imagine yourself lithe and slender in a new swimsuit or managing a thriving, demanding business, it could mean you have a self-esteem problem. Through age regression, hypnoanalysis can help you discover and deal with the event or relationship that resulted in your present lack of self-confidence. You may have lost confidence in yourself because relationships or events at some time in your life have battered your self-esteem. Your subconscious may harbor memories of such experiences. This was the case with Lindsay, who came to my office searching for "inner peace, for an end to the war that was going on inside me."

Her Self-esteem Was in the Gutter

Here's how Lindsay tells it:

> My self-esteem was in the gutter from a newly broken relationship. I had failed at my business. My children had been admitted to an adolescent psychiatric ward for emotional disturbance. I was 50 pounds overweight. My life was a mess!

When she first came in, Lindsay ranked her problems at 10 on a severity scale of 1 to 10. By the time she gave the above evaluation, she was still involved in a therapy group but indicated she thought her problems were at a three level. As I worked with her, I determined that Lindsay was in a spiritual depression. She approached just about every aspect of her life from a negative perspective. Read her further comments and see whether you agree.

> The war inside me is slowly coming to a close, my self-esteem is no longer at the bottom of the barrel all the time—maybe 25 percent of the time. I have a very good job with tremendous potential. My oldest daughter is doing much better, but the younger one is still struggling.
>
> My hypnoanalytic process has been a truly rewarding experience. I gave a part of me in the history and word-association tests that no one ever knew. In fact the history and word tests were revealing to me as well.
>
> After the initial, face-to-face history, my journey into hypnosis began. We regressed back to being in the womb, allowing me to let go of certain issues associated with my birth. The death suggestion I had carried around most of my life was incredible. Little by little, Ryan has helped me peel away layers of problems. As issues came up, his awareness and intuitiveness allowed me to deal with them and let them go.
>
> My therapy has helped, changed, and affected me in many very positive ways. My overall disposition is better. I am able to work through problems as they arise. I've lost 40 pounds. I've increased my income and continue to receive good performance reviews with offers of other jobs within my company. My relationship with my daughters has improved. I'm able to talk with my former husband. And, my opinion of myself has gone from 0 to a 9, with 10 being the highest.
>
> I now look forward to all the endless possibilities that my life has in store for me—I should say, "for the new me."

RE-IMAGING CAN HELP SOLVE PROBLEMS

Some of the suggestions I gave Lindsay under hypnosis helped with re-imaging. She was having trouble with positive imagery. Her self-esteem had ebbed below the point necessary for personal respect, and having lost respect for herself, she could not image herself with value. She was in a self-defeating cycle.

Here are some suggestions I give clients to help in re-imaging:

1. Shell out negative images. Identify your negative self-images and put them aside. What is stopping you from succeeding? Anything other than lack of knowledge or experience is a self-imposed limitation. Learning is available, and so is experience. Assuming that you are not sufficiently attractive, bright, talented, organized, or energetic to succeed is self-sabotage.

2. Re-image. See and feel yourself in opposite situations. This game requires you to see your desired life-style in the future. Assume that you will face no obstacles in achieving your desired situation. Simply expect that you will be able to devote your full attention to reaching your goals. See yourself as you want to be. Your route to the goal will be easier if your imagery is not fraught with self-doubts and "what-ifs."

You have the opportunity, through the process of personal renewal and re-imaging, to discover limitless adventure. The key to that adventure is within you, but you can only open the door if you are willing to accept new challenges and peer into unexplored horizons of change and growth.

Some people feel afraid of new experiences, even if their old ones are destructive or provide bad feelings. With some people, it's as if they don't know they're alive unless they feel bad.[3]

KEEP IMAGERY STATEMENTS POSITIVE

The power of visualization lies in the quality of your images. Your programming statements must be positive to achieve positive results. If you cannot imagine a situation, you will have difficulty achieving it. By the same token, the stronger the feelings attached to the imagery of something you desire, the better your chances of reaching it.

Use mime imagination to bring your images into the here and now. When you put yourself into a scene, take all your senses with you. Let your imagination create for you the sights, sounds, feelings, and smells of the reality you desire.

Self-affirmation statements are the core of conscious activity in reprogramming your subconscious. Keep these rules in mind when planning your reprogramming:

1. Self-affirmations must be in the present tense. Since the subconscious deals only with the present, keep your affirmations in that tense. For example, don't pledge, "I *will* get up early tomorrow." Affirm instead, "I enjoy getting up early."

2. Keep self-affirmations in the first person. Your subconscious has no control over anyone or anything except you and your actions. Say, "I enjoy being productive at work and my efforts reward me more and more" or something similar, not, "I *will* get a raise at work."

Your subconscious does not have the power to guarantee that you actually receive a raise. It can only be used to improve your productivity, thereby, leading to a raise. However, your subconscious can draw circumstances to you to improve your situation.

3. Brief self-affirmations are more effective. The subconscious can accept short (seven words or less) affirmations easier than it can accept lengthy, verbose intellectualizations.

4. Repeat self-affirmations frequently. To assure that self-affirmations become rooted in the subconscious, repeat them at least seven times, pausing between each repetition.

5. Visualize success while programming your mind. Visualization without emotional backing is less powerful than when it is propelled by powerful feelings.

6. Image success from two perspectives. "See" your images both as a spectator and as a participant. Visualize yourself receiving the award as "best whatever" of the year and see yourself from the view of someone in the audience. Use kinesthetic and auditory imagination. Hear the applause as you step up to receive the award. Feel the solid weight of the plaque or the smooth curvature of the loving cup as you take it into your hands.

7. Never visualize failure. Many unsuccessful persons focus on a negative result. "What am I going to do if I don't win?" The subconscious is attracted to its images—either positive or negative. Fear produces that which one is afraid of. Visualizing success is necessary for a positive outcome in any endeavor. Say no to fear.

SLEEP LEARNING ALSO EFFECTS CHANGE

I said earlier that effective visualizing occurs when our brains are in the alpha state. The alpha state can also be a doorway to learning. As you slip from the wakeful state into light sleep, you enter a state in which the conscious mind is relaxed and the subconscious mind is ready to absorb new information and ideas. Thomas Budzynski, Ph.D., calls this the "twilight zone."

Budzynski and his colleagues at the Biofeedback Institute of Denver conducted research into sleep learning during the 1970s. They found that as individuals fall asleep they go from "a relaxed alpha brain-wave pattern, accompanied by slow, rolling eye movements, to the disappearance of alpha and its replacement by slower, small-amplitude theta waves . . . within roughly five to 10 minutes."[4] During this brief period in which the mind drifts from the alpha state into the theta state, "people not only may have creative insights but may also be more in touch with the unconscious in general. They are hyper-suggestible and capable of learning certain things more efficiently and painlessly than during the day when logical and analytical factors are in control."[5]

Arthur Koestler explained it this way:

> The temporary relinquishing of conscious controls liberates the mind from certain constraints which are necessary to maintain the disciplined routines of thought but may become an impediment to the creative leap. At the same time, other ideas of ideation on more primitive levels of mental organization are brought into activity.[6]

Adds Budzynski:

> The twilight state, I believe, opens a kind of pipeline to the unconscious, to the non-rational half of our brain that we usually ignore. If we learn to open the pipeline at will, rather than by chance, perhaps we can resolve some of the conflicts between the conscious and unconscious mind—conflicts that create problems in many areas of our lives.[7]

Budzynski's "twilight state" and Koestler's "temporary relinquishing of conscious controls" are both characteristics of hypnosis. Hence, a person can be taught, through self-hypnosis, to achieve at will the state of consciousness in which sleep learning can take place.

In recent decades, sleep learning has become a popular method of assimilating information or influencing behavior. Athletes use it before performances. Students use it to learn course material. Doctors use it to assist patients in overcoming illness. Parents use it to direct positive results in their children.

Dr. Leo Martello gathered several well-known examples of successful sleep learning for his article in *The New Journal of Hypnotism*:[8]

- Through sleep learning, entertainer Art Linkletter picked up enough of the Mandarin Chinese language in 10 days to carry on a televised conversation with the vice-consul of Nationalist China.
- A reporter for *Mechanics Illustrated* studied Spanish in her sleep for seven nights. After the experience, she was able to read books and carry on a conversation in the language.
- A high-school graduate passed the examinations for a four-year college course following nine months of sleep learning.

- Branches of the U.S. armed forces taught servicemen Morse Code using sleep-learning methods.

"The subconscious mind itself never sleeps and has a perfect memory," writes Martello. "In our competitive society, tensions are part of our everyday living; yet sleep learning has been a boon to people suffering from frustrations, tensions, inability to relax or sleep well, and other complaints which prevent one from making the most of his inner resources."[9]

THE PREHYPNOTIC SUGGESTION

There's an easy and simple way to program positive attitudes into your subconscious. I call it the prehypnotic suggestion. You can do it with a simple exercise just before you go to sleep and just after waking, when your subconscious is most open to suggestion and you're actually in a hypnotic state or moving into one.

Take a blank sheet of ordinary paper and write on it a positive suggestion. For example, you might write, "Nobody on the staff is a better salesperson than I am. I am going to prove it during this sales campaign by winning that trip to the Bahamas."

Having written down the suggestion, fold the paper in half, covering what you have written. Keep it by your bed. When you first wake up in the morning, open it and read it three times. Do the same thing just before you fall asleep at night. Do this for 30 days and see what happens.[10] (You may want to write one suggestion for morning and one for evening. You can do that by writing on both sides of the paper.)

The more sensory data you give the subconscious mind through the suggestion, the more effective the suggestion. See yourself impeccably groomed, wearing your most potent power suit, giving a flawless presentation to a major client. Visualize the lines on the sales chart climbing steadily upward. See yourself on the deck of the cruise ship, inhaling the ocean air, or sipping a tropical drink beneath gently swaying palm trees, or dancing to marimba music with someone you love (or could love). Hear the music of the marimba band, or the drone of the surf massaging the shore. Feel the warm tropic breeze against your face. Taste the tangy sweetness of the drink and feel the lazy, warm glow from the rum.

Another technique is to involve a partner in the suggestion process. Make a deal with your spouse or someone else close to you. Have your partner repeat the suggestion to you just before you go to sleep and again in the morning after you wake up. Your spouse could whisper into your ear as you're drifting off to sleep, "I love you. You are on your way to winning that sales contest and we're going to the Caribbean."[11]

You may not want to ask anyone to repeat the same message to you every morning and every night for 30 days. So there's a simple alternative: Get the suggestion on tape. Have your partner record it so that you can play it each night upon retiring and each morning before arising. Or ask your friends or relatives to put the same suggestion or a related one on the same tape and finish the tape off by giving yourself all the positive affirmations and suggestions you'd like.

As you can see, self-hypnosis is not some supernatural state in which you walk around like a robot. It's as natural as falling asleep and waking up. When you are in this state, your subconscious has its ears open, awaiting suggestions from you. You can take advantage of this openness by making sure that your subconscious hears only positive suggestions, for the suggestions it hears are the suggestions it will act upon. Keep them positive.

Here are three books to further help you with relaxation or self hypnosis:

You Can't Afford the Luxury of a Negative Thought
A book for people with any life-threatening illness—including life.
John Roger & Peter McWilliams
(Prelude Press, 1988, 1989)

Peace, Love, & Healing
Body-mind communication and the path to self-healing: an exploration.
Bernie S. Siegel, M.D.
(Walker & Co., 1990)

You Can Heal Your Life
Louis L. Hay
(Hay House, Inc., 1984)

Key Concepts

- Relaxation is the key to reprogramming and self-hypnosis, the key that opens the door to taking control of our attitudes, our behavior, and the stress in our lives.
- You can utilize the processes of relaxation, self-hypnosis, imagery, and sleep learning to boost your self-esteem and to program whatever you want into your mind.
- You can condition yourself to go into a deep-breathing, relaxed state by adopting a cue and repeating it as you achieve relaxation.
- The subconscious does not recognize the difference between fantasy and reality. You can be what you imagine, believe, and feel to be true.
- Self-affirmation statements are the core of conscious activity in reprogramming your subconscious.
- The power of imagery lies in the emotional quality of your images.

Growth Exercise

1. Recognize that your subconscious can heal your life.
2. Organize three positive suggestions, using your imaging power that will be very powerful in your life from this time on.
   a.
   b.
   c.
3. "Y.E.S." For the remainder of your life, maintain an attitude of YES. Say yes to health, wealth, happiness.
4. Consider the following affirmation as yours for all time: "I am willing to release the pattern within me that has caused this condition or experience—I accept responsibility and build only good things in my life."
   —Contributed by Dr. Roy Johnson, M.D.

CHAPTER SEVEN

SURVIVING WITHOUT SMOKING

A bad habit is at first a caller,
then a guest,
and at last a master.

—Anonymous

UNCONTROLLED SUBSTANCE ABUSE

Mark Twain said: "Stopping smoking is easy. I have done it a thousand times." It's a lament heard far too often.

Tobacco is one of the three most abused chemical substances in our society. Alcohol and coffee are the others. A large percentage of America's health-care dollar is spent treating conditions caused by use of these substances.

Smoking is not only a physical addiction and a bad habit, but, more importantly, it's an emotional attachment—an addictive relationship that can be very disquieting to let go of. Research shows that smoking permanently destroys air sacs in the lungs. Every drag on a cigarette irritates and changes cells and lung tissue.

The American Cancer Society has put together a list of more than 80 reasons to stop smoking, including the dangers from cancer, heart attack, stroke, emphysema, bronchitis, poor circulation, poor coordination and vision, coughing, clogged and black lungs, slowed reflexes, reduced endurance, more frequent colds, influenza and pneumonia, miscarriages, wrinkles, and asthmatic attacks. Actually, the research links smoking with more and more physical problems as each year goes by.

The late chest surgeon Dr. Harold Levin added to the case against smoking. Levin reported that a one-pack-a-day smoker destroys 1 percent of his lungs each year. Lung cancer is not reversible. Most lung-cancer victims will be dead within six to nine months; 1 out of 5 will survive one year, and 1 out of 10 will be dead within five years. All end up with lung disability.

Pointing to the effects of nicotine, former U.S. Surgeon General C. Everett Koop contended that cigarettes were as addictive as cocaine or heroin. My experience with addicted persons supports Koop's conclusion, but more from a subconscious psychological or emotional perspective than from a strictly physical dependence on nicotine. It's what smoking means for the smoker's emotions and in his or her subconscious that really counts. Falling in love is a powerful stimulant on many levels. Smoking is also a powerful stimulant, except that the smoker may fall in love with the grim reaper so to speak.

KNOWLEDGE AND AWARENESS HAVE INCREASED

After the surgeon general's statement became public, I started receiving more calls at my office from smoking-cessation seekers. As a result of that influx of calls, I collected a fair amount of data describing the love affair many people have with cigarettes. "They're my only friend," one lonely widow said. "I don't know what I'd do with my hands if I quit," quipped a celibate smoker. "I'm mad at myself for being controlled by a long, thin, white thing," said one person.

These examples illustrate my point that an emotional bonding takes place between cigarette and smoker. Why else would anybody continue such a slow-motion suicidal behavior with so many harmful side effects, unless the person is crazy, which usually isn't the case?

SMOKING IS NOT LOVE, BUT HATE

Smoking is like getting mad at yourself. How is that? Well, smoking is a logical choice for someone who believes he or she is guilty of something and needs punishment.

During my treatment of smokers, I read to the client words and phrases such as:

Punishment.
The reason I smoke is . . .
My punishment is . . . .

In 40 percent to 50 percent of the people I see, the responses under hypnosis to the word "punishment" are: "self," "guilt," "necessary," "hate," or "unavoidable." People rarely if ever respond positively to the thought "the reason I smoke is . . . " I get responses such as: "terrible," "no good reason," "nervousness," and "anxiety." Almost invariably, clients respond with "smoking" to the phrase "my punishment is . . ."

Smoking Was Her Security Blanket

We punish ourselves for the strangest reasons. I had a client named Sally who punished herself because she was adopted. Once she realized what she was doing, she gave up smoking easily and has remained cigarette-free ever since—four years as of this writing. Sally came to my office saying she guessed she was finally ready to give up smoking. She told me:

> I've been battling it for a long time. I just think I need emotional reinforcement. I quit once for a whole year after I had surgery, but I began again after I broke up with somebody about 15 years ago.

Both her parents and several other people in her family smoked. Sally originally started smoking at 16 (thought she looked "cool" smoking and everyone was doing it), gave it up at 40, resumed the habit at 41, and was 56 years old when she came to me. Realizing that her taking up smoking at 16 when she "thought I looked 'cool' and everyone was doing it" was a symptom-producing event, I asked why she considered smoking a problem.

> It's just an emotional crutch with me. I use them as oral gratification. Whenever I get emotionally upset, I reach for a cigarette. I want to be healthier again. I smoke a good pack a day.

I asked her about traumatic events in her life.

> A friend died recently—a heart attack in his sleep. He was 68. We had broken up the previous year, but there was still a lot of anger.

The friend's death turned out to be a symptom-intensifying event. Searching in her background for other traumatic events, she said her parents had died 22 years earlier—within four days of each other. This event is a big death suggestion. As I plowed further into her history, I found additional death suggestions:

> My surgery 15 years ago, chest and breast. There was a possibility of cancer, but I came out clean. I had pneumonia and nearly died at six years old. . . . Oh God, I don't remember . . . whooping cough as a child, a baby. I had my tonsils out [she looked to heaven] in second grade. My nose had to be operated on twice to breathe. The second time they straightened it out, I was about 18. Somebody held me under water at 12 or 13. I had a D&C about 10 years ago. I never got married.

Then came the information we'd been searching for: the initial sensitizing event.

> I was adopted. I didn't know about it 'til I was 16 years old. My parents never intended to tell me.

That was the key. Her adoption was the initial sensitizing event; learning about it was a symptom-producing event. She had started smoking when she found out she was adopted, and she had had all those death suggestions: the pneumonia, the tonsils, the whooping cough, the nose jobs, the near-drowning.

During her word-association test, in response to my phrase "If I were happy . . ." Sally said "I would stop smoking." When I said, "I punish myself . . ." she said, "Because I don't think I am good enough because I am adopted." She also said she started smoking because she thought it would be "sexy."

Once we reviewed her history and word-association test she decided to leave smoking in the past. She realized she was filling in some empty space. She was suffering from both spiritual and physical walking-zombie syndromes.

In Sally's subconscious mind, smoking proved that she was indeed alive spiritually and emotionally. She filled in the empty spaces inside her by smoking, too. She agreed that what she needed was not smoke, or self-punishment, but love and caring and the companionship of other people. As a result of this awareness, she agreed to stop smoking, to stop punishing herself, and to seek out those particular gratifications that she needed, namely to bring her self-love back to life.

Sally left cigarettes in the past. She did not even come in for her sixth session. She felt so good about her progress that she called me a year later to thank me again for helping her understand her problem.

REASONS FOR SMOKING

There's a lot more going on within a person who smokes than merely the development of a physical addiction or a bad habit. There frequently are serious underlying reasons for their behavior enclosed within their subconscious minds. It's those reasons that I uncover during hypnoanalysis. The key to success in therapy is enabling clients to understand how their misinterpretations of reality caused them to smoke as a way of surviving a particular event. By smoking, Sally punished herself for her "unworthiness" resulting from having been adopted. And following all those scrapes with death when she felt she could not breathe, she proved she was alive by seeing the smoke (breath) coming from her lungs.

He Was a Chain Smoker

Philip M. Bonelli shared a classic survival example in the *Journal of Medical Hypnoanalysis.*[1]

> My favorite case is a 55-year-old ex-Marine who had been smoking four packs of cigarettes a day. When he came into therapy, after taking a detailed history, it became apparent that this individual did not begin smoking until he was on a Pacific island during the Second World War. One day enemy aircraft were strafing the island. He was crouching in a foxhole with another Marine, frightened for his life. At that point the other Marine offered him a cigarette saying, in effect, that if he smoked the cigarette, he would feel better, that is, he would be safe. In a moment of high emotional energy (trauma) my patient smoked the cigarette, making the subconscious survival association that if he did smoke he would feel better, or in other words, he would survive. He smoked the cigarette and he survived that particular attack. Thereafter, each time there was an enemy attack he lit a cigarette believing, subconsciously, that by smoking the cigarette he would be ok. The result was that he did survive. [But his survival had nothing to do with his smoking.] This, of course, reinforced his whole subconscious concept that if he smoked he would live. Subsequently, he got out of the war without a scratch, but smoking four packs of cigarettes a day.

TRUTH OR MYTH?

It's important to separate the truth from myths about smoking. Smoking is not just an addiction to nicotine; it is much more than a simple addiction. Smoking is not something one does for pleasure, though people claim so; it is a very dangerous habit. Smoking is not only a physical addiction and a bad habit; it is also an emotional attachment, an investment of energy in a deadly behavior. It isn't the physical dependence on nicotine that keeps smokers from quitting. What smoking represents in the subconscious is what really prevents them from stopping successfully.

Smokers get what they expect. If they expect relaxation, they get relaxation; if they expect to be energized, they get a spurt of energy; if they expect sexual stimulation, they feel it. Nicotine, however, is a stimulant not a relaxant, and smoking can actually inhibit sexual performance and endurance due to decreased blood flow.

Dr. Ellen Langer substantiated the mind-body theory in recent research at Harvard University. In work that won her the Distinguished Contributors to Psychology in the Public Interest Award from the American Psychological Association, Langer compared the mindful and mindless approaches to dealing with addictions such as smoking or alcohol abuse.

She found that smokers in nonsmoking environments did not experience strong cravings for cigarettes. They could forgo their habits in a movie theater, at work, or during religious holidays (Orthodox Jews are not permitted to smoke on the Sabbath). When the same individuals returned to settings where smoking was allowed, however, they experienced withdrawal symptoms if they could not smoke. On smoke breaks at work, for instance, the craving returned.

Admitting that this phenomenon occurred mindlessly, Langer and her students then designed an experiment to determine whether the same effect could be achieved mindfully—in other words, whether people could control the experience of temptation. She reports:

> In designing a second experiment to answer this question, we assumed that a mindful person would look at addiction from more than one perspective. For instance, it is clear that there are actually advantages as well as disadvantages to addictions. But this is not the usual point of view of someone trying to break a habit.
>
> People who want to stop smoking usually remind themselves of the health risks, the bad smell, the cost, others' reactions to their smoking—the drawbacks of smoking. But these effects are not the reasons they smoke, so trying to quit for those reasons alone often leads to failure. The problem is that all of the *positive* aspects of smoking are still there and still have strong appeal—the relaxation, the concentration, the taste, the sociable quality of smoking.
>
> A more mindful approach would be to look carefully at these pleasures and find other, less harmful, ways of obtaining them. If the needs served by an addiction or habit can be satisfied in different ways, it should be easier to shake.[2]

Sally, in the earlier case study, agreed to find ways other than smoking to fill her personal acceptance and survival needs.

QUITTING IS DIFFERENT FOR EACH PERSON

We know from experience that stress builds up when someone tries to quit smoking. In issuing its recommendations for dealing with what it calls "the crazies," the American Cancer Society says: "Learn to relax quickly and deeply. Make yourself limp, visualize a soothing, pleasing situation, and get away from it all for a moment. Concentrate on that peaceful image and nothing else." Relaxation and visualization—that is what I talked about in Chapter Six, and it's what happens during the first session when patients come into my office for therapy to stop smoking.

The first step is an initial consultation and taking of history. Then, as the patient—wearing headsets and a blindfold—reclines in a comfortable lounge chair in a private room, I will be in a nearby control room where I will gently guide him or her into a state of relaxation. And relaxation, basically, encourages hypnosis. It's a very natural state of mind, which opens the door to the subconscious. During hypnosis, the conscious mind retreats and the subconscious mind becomes superconcentrated. By communicating with the subconscious, I'm able to uncover the underlying reasons for smoking. Then, in subsequent sessions, I deal with those reasons and resolve them. Once the causes are removed, patients no longer feel the need to continue smoking.

The Europes Both Quit

One of my most interesting experiences involves a retired couple who both came into the office for help in quitting smoking. I'll call them Mr. and Mrs. Europe. Mrs. Europe was a 55-year-old retired woman, born in Germany.

I walked in and said, "Are you ready to quit smoking?" and she said, "Yeah!"

I asked, "What's the problem?"

She responded, "I enjoy it; that's the big problem. I really enjoy it, but you come to the point where you wake up hacking. My chest is tight. I don't get over colds. I've tried three times to quit smoking."

I inquired, "Why do you consider smoking to be a problem?" and she said, "It takes a lot of time away from my precious time."

Now, that was interesting. She was older and she considered her remaining time precious. But that was a suspicion, and I had to investigate deeper to find out exactly what she meant. She said she'd been smoking about 30 years and usually had two packs a day, so I asked when she had started.

> I was a waitress, about 19 years old. I came over to the United States in 1949. I thought it was cool. I was just learning the language and I was young and dumb.

I asked about traumatic incidences in her life.

> "The war. Children dying from typhoid fever and malnutrition. I couldn't stomach the shooting of guns. When I was nine years old, in Germany,

> both my aunt and uncle were killed and my father was taken to Siberia for a year and a half.

Then she continued with a host of traumatic events.

> I lived with the Russian officers and saw rapes at eight or nine. I had diphtheria at seven. The thing to do then was to send people sick with diphtheria to a camp. I was in that hospital for seven weeks. My father was sort of an alcoholic and beat my mom, but that was nothing new. It was standard behavior in Old Europe.

She also reported that she had had a hysterectomy at age 34. And, here's an interesting point. I asked her when she got married. She had married Mr. Europe at 19—just before she began smoking.

I then asked her what she could do when she quit smoking that she could not do now. She said, "Oh, I'll have more time." Subconsciously, she was probably talking about more time to be alive, more time on the planet.

The remarkable thing about Mrs. Europe's case was that her smoking revolved around her coming to the United States—leaving her family, going through the traumatic events in World War II, and getting married. All those things happened within a few years. She started smoking while she was learning the language. It was a way of being connected, a way of proving that she was accepted in America.

In her word-association test, I said, "I'm just like . . ." She answered, "My dad." Her father, of course, had been dead for many years. Under hypnosis, I lined up all the traumatic events she had experienced as death suggestions: She had seen people die and others raped. She had left her home and given up her family. She had been alone. Her homeland had died so far as she was concerned.

She had met her husband and got married, and smoking had just seemed the thing to do. However, as is typical with people experiencing the walking-zombie syndrome, smoking proved to her subconscious mind that she was really alive.

Once I explained all that to her, she agreed with it and also agreed to stop smoking. So I gave her positive suggestions.

In a subsequent session, she came in saying, "I'm doing terrific. Not a one. So far, this has been so easy. I found two in the medicine cabinet and broke them up. How could people smoke!" After smoking for 30 years, she did not even experience withdrawal symptoms.

A year later, she called, reiterating how helpful the positive suggestions had been and how easy it had been for her to quit after she understood the reasons she smoked.

Mr. Europe's Case Was Very Different

Retired, 63-year-old Mr. Europe had been born in Poland and had come to this country when he was six or seven years old. When he came in, I asked him if he was ready to quit smoking and he said, "Yeah, I think it's time to give it up." I asked, "What's the problem?" and he responded:

> It seems like you are rewarding yourself for anything you do. You get nervous; anxious; you want to light up a cigarette. It's a reward. You are rewarding yourself and it makes you feel good.

So, I asked, "Why do you consider smoking to be a problem?" His reply was very revealing:

> You think you are going to die if you don't have one. You've always got to have that pack hidden somewhere.

Within the first few sentences, this man had told me that cigarettes were proving he was alive. His reason for smoking was similar to his wife's in some respects. Both had walking-zombie syndrome. Mrs. Europe had had many death suggestions, and smoking cigarettes was proof that she was alive, but her problems were more generalized. Her death suggestions were directed to her spirit, her body, her mind, and her country, among other things.

He had started smoking in high school. "The other kids were smoking," he said. "We used to sneak one."

He had said that he rewarded himself with cigarettes, that when he was 16 he would go sneaking one. He was still doing that as an adult, but it was also proof that he was alive. I asked Mr. Europe why he wanted to give up smoking, and he said, "I don't want to die from it, that's for sure." Let's pursue his subconscious thinking further under hypnosis through the word-association test:

Ryan: Because you think you're going to die if you don't . . .
Client: Quit smoking.
Ryan: When I started smoking . . .
Client: I felt big.

The last statement subconsciously signified his maleness. Now, there is a sign that he was proving that he was alive in his mind. His psychological "like" was connected to his smoking and being grown up. At age 16, there was another element to this man's story.

In the word-association test, many different factors will show up that would not normally be revealed if I were simply to trust the history and what a person says. For example:

Ryan: Anxiety, feels like . . .
Client: Excitement. (I had asked earlier what conditions influenced his smoking and he said that anxiety brought it on.)
Ryan: Smoking serves as a defense against . . .
Client: Tension.
Ryan: Tension feels like . . .
Client: Anxiety.
Ryan: Excitement feels like . . .
Client: To be aroused.
Ryan: Stimulate?
Client: Arouse.

Already, I was beginning to get a sense that smoking for him was a sexual substitute as well as proof that he was alive. One way he kept his sexuality alive when he was growing up was to smoke. He felt big when he smoked. All his responses were connected.

Under hypnosis, when I explained to him about his keeping himself alive, being big, and the connection to sexuality, he understood it and agreed with it. He said that he was definitely more interested in sexual activity than his wife was, and that he could understand how smoking could be a sexual substitute. After all the mouth is not only used for smoking, eating, and talking, but also in sex; and teenage boys are normally very sexual.

I always ask the client to have a dream about the problem he or she is trying to solve. Mr. Europe's dream further confirmed the sexual connection to his smoking when we wove the threads together in the subconscious mind. He dreamed he was installing and connecting waterproof boxes, under water, waist deep.

Installing and connecting are both words that reflect sexual imagery. Also the dream's setting—waist deep under water—suggests sexuality. We discussed the threads of a sexual component running through his history and his word-association test, and the meaning of the dream was clear to him.

Through her smoking, Mrs. Europe had been proving that she was alive, but it was different for him. Her case was spiritual—loss of love in several areas. His was clearly a case of sexual substitution that had begun when he was a teenager trying to prove that he was a man. Once we talked it over, he let go of his smoking and, I assume, took a deeper interest in his sexuality, as I had suggested.

These are only two of the many different themes or variables that we often identify as causes for someone's smoking. The reasons are unique to each person because of their experiences. Individuals react to and interpret their experiences in unique ways corresponding to their private logic.

My job is to help people come to terms with their streams of connectedness, with the order of survival in the subconscious. Smoking is almost always tied to a person's survival. Although a smoker's behavior does not make conscious sense, smoking can have a deep subconscious connection to survival either of one's mind, body, spirit, sexuality, or territory (see Chapter One on the order of importance for these forms of survival).

HYPNOSIS PROVIDES ACCESS TO THE SUBCONSCIOUS

Through hypnosis, greater access to subconscious attitudes and feelings that are responsible for behavior becomes available. It's possible to improve behavior and turn weaknesses into strengths by using gentle suggestions to help remove limiting beliefs and construct positive, life-affirming ones. However, the client must want to change. Hypnosis will not work unless it is accepted and wanted.

First, the underlying subconscious root causes of the emotional need for smoking are identified, analyzed, resolved, and removed. Then, when a person is free to give up the need for smoking, hypnosis techniques are used to remove the unwanted smoking habit pattern. This is the treatment of choice for the heavy smoker who has been unable to stop with other methods due to strong emotional need and attachment to smoking. Self-hypnosis is taught for easy, natural, and effective withdrawal to safeguard against substitution of other unwanted habits and to develop the ability to relax with mental imagery, improve health, breathe easier, and achieve more successful results generally.

The success rate in my simple, six-visit smoking cessation plan is 80 percent to 90 percent. No shots or drugs are used. I simply remove the subconscious motivation to smoke and create habit reformation. Best of all, hypnosis feels good. And I feel good, being an ex-smoker myself who quit cold turkey 17 years ago after going through hell year. Nobody has to feel withdrawal symptoms. I wish I had known of a hypnoanalyst at the time.

BENEFITS OF QUITTING SMOKING

If you're a smoker and decide to quit, you can expect positive changes to occur in your body as early as 20 minutes after you stop smoking. Consider these facts. Within 20 minutes after your last cigarette:

- Your blood pressure will decrease to your normal reading.
- Your pulse rate (heart beat) will decrease to normal for you.
- The temperature of your hands and feet will increase to its normal level.

It's never too late to stop. People who stop smoking after years of addiction still reduce their risk of coronary heart disease, according to a Yale University study which examined 2,674 smokers and former smokers between 65 and 74 years of age. The research indicated that the ex-smokers had 52 percent less risk of heart disease than those who continued smoking.[3] Here are some other physical changes you can expect after you've quit smoking:

- Within eight hours after your last cigarette, your blood's carbon-monoxide level will decrease to the normal amount and your blood will carry the normal amount of oxygen.
- Twenty-four hours after you quit smoking, your chances of a heart attack will decrease.
- Within 72 hours, the bronchial cilia will start to grow back and you'll begin to smell and taste things better.
- Three days after you stop smoking completely, your bronchial tubes will start to relax. You'll begin to breathe better, air will come in easier, and your lung capacity will increase.

Within 5 days, you can expect to experience the following:

- You will stop coughing.
- You will feel and sleep better.
- Your endurance will be increased.
- You will have more energy.
- You will digest food better.

- Your circulation will improve.
- Your coordination will be better.
- Your lungs will start to clear up.
- Your irritability level will decrease.
- You will enjoy life more and be proud of yourself.

Key Concepts

- Tobacco is one of the three most-abused chemical substances in our society.
- Smoking one pack a day will destroy 1 percent of your lungs each year.
- A lot more is going on in smokers' subconscious minds than merely the development of a physical addiction or a bad habit. Serious underlying reasons for their self-destructive behavior are enclosed within their subconscious minds.
- Smoking is not only a physical addiction and a bad habit; it is also an emotional attachment, an investment of energy in a deadly behavior.
- Smoking is nearly always tied to people's survival on one or more levels.
- My job in hypnoanalysis is to help people come to terms with their streams of connectedness, with the survival of the subconscious.
- Positive changes will begin to occur in your body as early as 20 minutes after you stop smoking.

Growth Exercise

Imagine you could trade smoking for something dear to you, something physical such as an arm, two legs, an eye, etc. In other words, what would you give up to continue smoking if you, hypothetically, were given a choice? ____

CHAPTER EIGHT

THE TROUBLE WITH FOOD IS: A FULL BODY IGNORES A HUNGRY SPIRIT

We are what we repeatedly do.
Excellence, then, is not an act, but a habit.

— *Aristotle*

Security is mostly a superstition.
It does not exist in nature. . . .
Life is either a daring adventure or nothing.

—*Helen Keller*

AND THE WEIGHT COMES BACK

Obesity is a complex matter involving psychological, physiological, and social components. Eating too much is a symptom and only part of the larger problem. Attempts to treat the symptoms alone usually result in failure and abandoned diets.

Diets don't work. A check of any magazine will reveal what most people know intuitively. If diets worked, there would not be the current glut of miraculous, doctor-sponsored, revolutionary, high-fiber, low-sodium, ad nauseum diets. If there really were a diet that worked, it would catch on and the market would dry up.

Diets fail because they do not address the real problem. People overeat for emotional reasons not because they like the taste of food. This fact is very difficult for overeaters to accept. Obesity, once it becomes entrenched, takes a considerable amount of effort to nullify because if the emotional attachment to overeating is not relieved, a cycle of consistent weight gain, guilt, dieting, and more weight gain begins. Along with the emotional and psychological component, the body gets accustomed to more weight and its set point (the weight at which the body feels comfortable) begins to rise, making weight loss more difficult. Add to this a slower metabolism, decreased activity, and the stimulation of the physical survival instinct by dieting[1] and you get obesity, depression, and hopelessness.

Recently, a weight-loss client came into my office with her eight-year-old daughter. The little girl sat down and announced: "My mom eats too much." This outspoken child, in her attempt to be helpful, thought she had identified the reason for her mother's visit. In her mind, her mother's overeating seemed straightforward enough. Like the child, many adults believe that weight problems stem simply from eating too much. The quantity of food a person eats doesn't begin to touch the complexity of eating disorders.

BEING OVERWEIGHT IS A HARD LIFE

Nearly all people with eating disturbances are negative thinkers. As a result of trying repeatedly and unsuccessfully to lose weight, their self-esteem plummets. They begin to think that, no matter how much they starve themselves and how hard they try, they cannot win the battle of the bulge.

They're right. Even if dieters succeed in taking off excess pounds, they usually regain the weight when they resume more normal eating and activity habits. Often, they end up weighing more than they did before they started dieting.

Although it is a step in the right direction, jumping into a busy exercise program is not the answer either. Exercise alone is neither efficient nor effective in reducing weight. Without positive eating habits, exercise is at best a temporary method of getting rid of excess fat. Regardless of how much you exercise, you will not lose weight if your body takes in more calories than it burns. People with weight problems must adopt and practice eating and exercise routines that support them in maintaining the weight that is normal for them.

An emotional attachment to food motivates people with obesity and eating disorders. It's not just a case of too little information or not enough motivation. Therefore, it is absolutely essential that weight control be attacked on at least three fronts:

- Psychological/emotional issues
- Eating habits
- Activity levels

It's been my experience that some people will accept eating and activity modifications but will resist all efforts at psychological or emotional interpretation. Experimenting with every fad diet that comes along, many end up despairing of the whole idea and growing increasingly despondent and fat. This is unfortunate because help is very much available.

The reason for failure, in part, has to do with the nature of psychological/emotional treatment and an innate sense of wanting to be right about ourselves and in control. Richard, one of my weight-loss clients, had been the victim of a very controlling parent. As he grew up, Richard learned he could control what he ate, as well as other bodily functions. Therefore, as a rebellious act, overeating became identified with his self-esteem. This case took a great deal of therapy, but his problem was finally resolved.

Psychological issues revolve around our beliefs and attitudes about ourselves, others, and the world in general. Woven inside the fabric of our beliefs lies our basic instinct, survival. Surviving is most important—our number-one concern. To be a human being means to survive. The survival instinct operates in three dimensions: mind, body, and spirit.

Perceived threats to our survival may be dealt with by overeating, resulting in obesity; by refusing to eat, resulting in anorexia; or by such behavior as going on eating binges, purging (bulimia), or other self-destructive actions. Unless the underlying negative suggestion to the person's survival is removed, all the dieting and food management will be counteracted by the will to survive. If, in the subconscious minds of overweight people, staying alive is associated with overeating, then what happens when they diet? Right, they feel like they are going to die.

The following case is an interesting example of a client whose weight problems stemmed from prebirth threats to her survival.

She Saw Herself Clearly

Barbara came into the office and my secretary asked her name. She said her real name but immediately amended it to "Fred Flintstone." Actually, she did look a little like Fred. She was short and chubby.

I greeted her with my usual, "What's the problem?" and she said right off:

> Don't you know by now? I don't know. I have an idea. I think I'm afraid of being rejected.

Then she repeated herself before going on.

> I think I'm afraid of being rejected. I think the weight is a defense mechanism and a way not to deal with either. I feel like so many other things are gone, I can honestly say I feel content [except for concern about] the weight right now. And the weight comes down to a larger issue.

Barbara did not identify the "larger issue," so I asked how long her weight had been a problem.

> I've always dabbled with the weight since I was a kid. It really hit about eight years ago. I met this guy, Alex [fictitious name]. I was truly in love with him. Then, one day he trailed off into the distance.

I asked, "What do you want from me?" and she responded:

> I want, [pause] to feel more comfortable in relationships. I don't want to be terrified, to cling, and to be walked on.

I asked if there had been problems during her birth or when her mother was carrying her. She revealed that her mother had been told that she could never have children. Barbara was born more than six weeks prematurely.

Frequently, the premature baby emerges into a traumatic emotional context. The context can be the result of the baby's wanting to get out of the womb quickly. It can also result from the perception that the mother wishes to eject (read "reject") the fetus. In either case, the baby experiences trauma associated with its being in the womb. So Barbara had hit on the cause when she said that her weight came down to a larger issue.

When I regressed her to the prenatal experience, Barbara did, in fact, feel her mother not wanting her. It was a mutual consent that her mother wanted her out and that she would leave earlier than normal. As a result of that experience, she concluded that she was not really wanted.

Her problem was spiritual. Twice in the initial interview, she had said she "was afraid of being." As a result of that fear, she wasn't being; she had become a spiritual walking zombie. She had an identity problem stemming from the death suggestion to her spiritual component before birth. She felt as if she didn't belong in the world. If her own mother hadn't wanted her, then who would? That's the way the private logic goes.

Under hypnosis, I helped Barbara understand that her mother was having problems with the pregnancy that were not related directly to her. Her mother would have felt uncomfortable regardless of whom was in her womb. She was, therefore, able to let go of her feeling of rejection and stop overeating to "keep herself alive." The only time she felt "filled up" was when she was stuffed with food. This addictive behavior, however, didn't solve her existential emptiness.

The initial sensitizing event was her prenatal experience. The loss of her boyfriend was a symptom-intensifying event. All of her life, she had tried to fill up her emotional void, and upon taking her lover, felt she was at last complete. Once he rejected her, the pain became aggravated, and it was then she sought out therapy.

This particular client demonstrated several features in her personality that hypnoanalysts call a Ponce de Leon syndrome (emotional and psychological immaturity). For example, believing that another person can fill one's emptiness is a childlike fantasy. Unfortunately, this client stopped treatment before I could help her with those illusions, but she claimed a victory from her analysis.

Pam Felt Possessed by Food

Pam, a single, 43-year-old research analyst from a major insurance company, came into my office saying she was having trouble maintaining her weight loss. At 5'4" and 150 pounds, she had already regained 10 of the 30 pounds she had managed to lose and felt she was heading back to obesity.

She reported being overweight since age seven, when her family had moved. She had undergone a tonsillectomy during the same year. I knew from past experience that tonsillectomies frequently result in death suggestions. People who have had tonsillectomies with ether as an anesthetic never forget that experience. Commonly, we say that we put a sick or injured animal to sleep. Taking ether is often subconsciously felt to be like being put to death. The individual goes into the hospital and is gassed. All too often, victims of ether tonsillectomies smoke cigarettes to prove they are alive, or overeat to fill up the empty space that was created by the death suggestion of the anesthesia. Smoking or overeating are only symptom-producing events, however. It's the initial sensitizing event that I want to identify.

I asked Pam what she wanted from me and she said, "I want to get to a reasonable weight and stay there. I don't want to be possessed by food. I'm addicted to eating."

Analyzing history, dreams, and word-association responses is a Sherlock Holmesian search for clues. I am looking for the initial event, symptom-producing events, and, of course, the symptom-intensifying events. Mainly, I'm after the initial event, then the conditioning events that have caused the person to stall with the problem.

On the word-association test, the client answered "I don't know" to:

"The reason I am overweight . . . ,"
"If I knew, I would never be punished . . . ," and
"My punishment is . . ."

So all those equal each other, and being overweight has to do with something about punishing. Earlier, I had said the word "problem" and she had responded "none."

That response is typical of adolescent problem denial. I took this direction in the word-association test:

RYAN: I reward myself . . .
PAM: Often.
RYAN: When I'm thin . . .
PAM: I feel sexy.

Evidently, Pam was avoiding being sexy by being overweight. I just had to look a little further to find the reason for it.

RYAN: The one thing I need most, is . . .
PAM: Love.
RYAN: The love stopped when . . .
PAM: My mother died.

There was a hint that some of Pam's emptiness resulted from her relationship with her mother, and that she felt love had died when her mother did. Her mother also had a weight problem and died at 65 when Pam was in her early twenties.

RYAN: Instead of food, I'd really rather . . .
PAM: Make love.
RYAN: Because of the emptiness . . .
PAM: Feels horrible inside.

When I reviewed all my observations and explained to Pam that she had a spiritual walking-zombie syndrome, that her self-love had died, and that she was punishing herself, it made a lot of sense to her. She became eager to continue.

Throughout the weight-reduction program, which runs about 30 sessions, I gave her many suggestions about developing a strong self-image, about not being possessed by food, and about using food for fuel, not as a filler or a defense against other negative elements in her life.

The analysis of her assigned dream was helpful also. Reporting her dream, Pam wrote:

> It was very dark. I was confined in something very close to me, like a box. I was in an upright position and there was beating and scratching at the box. I made sounds, but I wasn't screaming. I had the feeling of suffocating. There was no one else in the dream. I woke up highly agitated, hot and sweating.

When I reviewed this dream—indicative of birth imagery, or prenatal experience—with Pam, she said:

> I was terrified I was dying. There was a part of me that wanted to get out, but I put a brick wall around myself.

Concluding that her overweight condition was a substitute for that safe, womblike experience, I decided to regress her to the time she was three months old intrauterine.

She talked about being confused about her father. She said her mother was very upset that her father would never be a good provider.

Pam reported that she had never wanted to be in the way in her family and had always worked hard to gain her parents' approval, even to the point of sacrificing herself. Here she was at 43. Never married. Although she was very attractive and appealing to many people, having had several affairs, she had never actually been able to grow past a childlike dependency on her parents. This was the Ponce de Leon syndrome in action.

In another session, I regressed her back to the womb and to birth. She said:

> It feels painful, awkward and I recognize it is going to be a change from security. I am afraid. It is different. It's wide open. I am insecure. Nothing close and secure to me.
>
> They wrapped me in a blanket to take me to the nursery. It feels like there is so much space, it's overwhelming. All these babies.

When she recognized that feeling of needing to be wrapped up, of needing to have something close to her, of security that was threatened by her birth, she was able to let go of the negative suggestions she had received from the birth event. Those suggestions were related to the protection she felt from her excess weight.

In this case, I dispensed with the other symptom-intensifying events and symptom-producing events. For once she and I discovered that feeling in the womb, Pam recognized how she was using food to achieve a sense of security. Pam eliminated elements of punishment and immaturity on her own and was no longer tied to the memories of her parents. After these sessions, she reported an increased ability to form secure and loving relationships with both men and women.

Weight cases are frequently very involved, with numerous elements contributing to the problem. Pam's case was fairly simple and straightforward. She has kept in touch with me over the years since her therapy and continually reports that she is doing very well. However, she still has to come to terms with the ups and downs of normal life.

PROBLEMS ARE NOT ALWAYS AS THEY APPEAR

From the preceding examples, you can understand how weight problems originate from an emotional-psychological-spiritual time warp and how obesity is only a symptom. For many, what, at face value, looks like the problem is in reality not the problem at all but a solution to an earlier problem.

Some weight-control programs urge people to associate something unpleasant with the foods they crave. For example, they are told to see chocolate bars as riddled with worms. If the root cause of overeating is not ferreted out and dealt with, if their self-image is not changed, some other food will just be substituted for the "wormy" chocolate bars, and the individuals will go right on maintaining their "survival" behavior.

HYPNOANALYSIS DISCOVERS THE CAUSE BEHIND THE CAUSE

Beliefs lodged in the subconscious, which have no basis in current fact, can control a person's eating patterns and behavior, resulting in the individual's being overweight or underweight. In my work as a hypnoanalyst, I have helped many people come to terms with the real reason behind their overeating. My comprehensive weight-loss program first identifies, then analyzes, resolves, and removes the underlying subconscious emotional and psychological causes for the need to overeat. Then, a medically managed weight-reduction food program is individually designed and prescribed, using hypnosis techniques to remove the undesirable faulty eating habits and related behavior problems.

Excess fat and inches come off easily and naturally, allowing for a permanent return to normal, lean weight levels through healthy, practical, positively controlled, sensible eating patterns, without the use of will power, medications, or starvation diets. My program emphasizes developing a positive mental attitude, an improved self-image, increased activity and energy levels, and a feeling of health and well-being—physically, mentally, emotionally, and spiritually.

The Case of Mrs. Processor

"What's the problem?" I asked the patient.

"Too much," replied Mrs. Processor.

It was obvious what she had "too much" of. The lady was overweight.

"I'm dieting forever," she told me. Her kids would tell her she was fat. She had lost weight several times, but each time she regained it. Her older brother also was "very large."

She told me she was suffering from depression. She had sold her house. Her parents had moved to Florida. She had lost a relative to death in the past year. She said she had a lot of "death suggestions" coming at her.

"What makes you feel better?" I asked.

"Spending money makes me feel better, and then I feel guilty. I feel good when I'm eating, and I feel guilty afterwards."

I asked what she would be able to do after being cured of these problems that she couldn't do before the cure.

She answered that she would like to get over the feeling of being ugly and "probably just feel better and be myself."

"What do you want from me?" I inquired.

"To get rid of all this. Basically, I'd like to lose weight and feel good about myself."

I did a counseling history with her and took her through many sessions. We seemed to be getting nowhere. She wanted to be put on the weight program, so I obliged.

I asked her what the problem was with her weight, and she said it was probably from not taking time to eat properly. Finally, toward the end of the 10th weight session, it came out: "Maybe I'm afraid of men."

I explored that comment with her.

"Back when I first got married, I didn't really date any men."

We went to the word-association test, and it went like this:

Ryan: My relationship to food reminds me of . . .
Mrs. P.: Sex.
Ryan: I really desire . . .
Mrs. P.: Food.

So in her subconscious mind, Mrs. Processor equated food with sex. Subconsciously, it was sex that she was really desiring.

We continued the word-association test.

Ryan: My fat serves me as a defense against . . .
Mrs. P.: Sex.
Ryan: Sex . . .
Mrs. P.: In bed.
Ryan: What I'm afraid of . . .
Mrs. P.: Being attractive. When I'm thin I'm afraid.
Ryan: Affair . . .
Mrs. P.: Scary.
Ryan: If I were thin, I'd be . . .
Mrs. P.: Sexy.
Ryan: I'm afraid when . . .
Mrs. P.: I'm alone.

It didn't require a clairvoyant to see that the underlying issue with Mrs. Processor was her desire for more sex.

How often did she have sex with her husband?

"Maybe three times a month."

How often would she like to have it?

"None. It's not the main thing in my life."

Was sex satisfying?

"To me, yeah, but not to him," she laughed.

When I explained to Mrs. Processor the relationship between her desire for sex and her problem with weight, she terminated the treatment.

"I don't think we're dealing with the right things," she said.

We were, in fact, dealing with the right things. I had done birth regressions and regressions to events in her past, but we never seemed to get anywhere. She never seemed to deal with the issue.

Her case demonstrates how people will sacrifice themselves to maintain something that's more important. (Remember the order of importance). Mrs. Processor was married. She didn't really want to leave her husband, even though their sex life was unsatisfactory. She was afraid that if she became thin and attractive she would want to have an affair. The affair would threaten something that was much more important to her—her connection to love, to her husband, and to her family.

Needless to say, she didn't have to do that. All she really had to do was to deal with the fear and with the fact that she wanted to have more sex. She could have dealt with her feelings and not have to act on her feelings.

It would be inaccurate to characterize Mrs. Processor's problem as a sexual issue. It looked like a sexual issue, but it was really a spiritual issue. She was sacrificing her body to maintain her spiritual connection, which had to do with love and her husband. She was willing to sacrifice her body to obesity, to stifle her sexual impulses, and to forgo sexual gratification to keep something more important—her relationship to her husband and family. How tragic that she could not be brought to realize that the sacrifices were not necessary.

Mrs. Processor's story is not all tragedy, though. She did undertake a number of changes in her life. I recently received a letter from her in which she told me how she was doing. She wrote:

> I've grown in several ways. One: I think more, which means I look at the situation first, think about it, and then my reaction is either helpful or meaningful. I don't react and then think about what I should have done or said or not eaten.
>
> I take more time for myself. I sew more, read, take walks, etc.
>
> I really try to think why I want to eat. Is it anger, hunger, or necessity?
>
> I've learned that I can't change what my parents do. I may not like it when they drink, but it's not my problem.

> [It] still is very difficult for me to determine why I eat. I really feel I'm trying to eat good things, but I haven't lost weight. I know I should write down what I'm eating during the day and that would help, but I don't do it. Some day I will.
>
> My relationship with my husband is better because we are talking more. I can tell him what's bothering me, and he's starting to tell me things that bother him. I feel we're getting better.

So all wasn't lost in this case. Mrs. Processor developed significant insight, and a quote from Dr. Bryan seems to the point: "Leave something to God."

EATING DISORDERS DO THREATEN SURVIVAL

Bulimia and anorexia nervosa are life-threatening disorders involving food. Obesity, depending on the amount of it, often presents a threat to a person's health. If it does, more than medical attention is needed because medical attention alone (or in conjunction with dieting or exercise) works only on the symptoms of the problem.

Through hypnosis, I regress eating-disorder patients to their childhood or prebirth experiences to discover the initial sensitizing event that set them up for destructive eating patterns. Through hypnoanalysis, they not only receive immediate relief from their life-threatening symptoms, but also achieve a permanent resolution of the problem. As simple as I make this sound, Herculean effort is often required of both the patient and me to effect a cure. The patient in these cases is really the hero or heroine because treatment can be frustrating and expensive, and at times patients feel that it's "two steps forward and one back."

She Was Searching on Every Side

Janice was seeing four other therapists and was suicidal when she came to my office suffering from anorexia, depression, and low self-esteem. I greeted her with, "What's the problem?" and she laid out a list that would overwhelm the most astute professional:

> Not liking myself. I feel beneath everybody.
>
> Making decisions. I can't make a decision. I think everything has to be perfect in what I do, or it makes me mad.

> Jealousy. I think that has to do with not liking myself. Growing up in an alcoholic environment, 'cause I was always made fun of a lot. My dad would make fun of me, then abuse me.
>
> The basic problem right now, though, is not liking myself.

I asked how long it had been a problem, and she said as far back as she could remember. When I asked what she would be able to do once she was cured that she could not do now, she said:

> Be alone. I don't like being alone because then I feel lost. Every once in a while I get an anxiety attack.

So, I asked about past traumas: accidents? deaths? illnesses? operations? problems in her sex life? She groaned, "Oh, God!" I concluded that her relationship with God was the most traumatic problem. God translates into love, for God is love. Then she went on with another overpowering list of negative events in her life:

> When I was a little girl, I watched this friend forced to take her clothes off in a stream, and I didn't do anything to help.
>
> My dad's drunkenness. My brother went away to school and left me alone at 12.
>
> My Aunt Emile died, and I was made to go up to her casket at age eight.
>
> Then my dad tried to drown my mother in a pool when I was a teenager.

Notice that all these traumatic things had to do with losses of love. An incest victim, the first loss was the love of herself. She cried when telling me about it. I asked about premarital intercourse and she said:

> All I remember was that I was real scared. My brother was going away to school and he wouldn't protect me any more. I was probably around 12 years old. It started at eight years old.

I asked if there was anything she hadn't told me that she thought I really should know and she responded:

> Just the fact that I'm not a very nice person. I'm jealous.

When I asked what she wanted from me, she said simply, "I guess that I'll like myself a lot better."

Janice was experiencing a spiritual problem. She felt self-loathing conditioned by her loss of love, experiences in the womb, and living in an alcoholic/abusive house.

Janice's womb regression revealed that her mother felt totally overwhelmed. Janice's father was actively drinking while abusing her mother, who questioned whether she could handle another child. The pregnancy was fraught with turmoil. Janice, being totally dependent on her mother, incorporated the negativity and, hence, was born with the feeling of being unwanted.

But there was more to her case. Janice was conditioned to feel as she did by the things that happened to her. People who experience sexual abuse carry a lot of guilt.

Janice's first sexual experience was at eight years of age, with her drunken father. Her words: With Dad in my bedroom. All I remember was that I was real scared. My brother was going away to school and he wouldn't protect me any more."

She complained of feeling seven years old frequently, and in a dream analysis identified the feeling that she stopped growing at eight and wished to get no older.

Janice's food disturbance was related to a time she recalled in regression. When she was 16, her father didn't want to have sex with her any more because of her weight. She decided that "food's bad for you." Consequently, when she felt rejected, her symptom was abstinence from food. In Janice's subconscious, the idea of getting approval was linked to being sexually desirable.

I do not want to oversimplify this case. It took a lot of courage on her part and a lot of work on the part of both of us. But it was well worth it. She is functioning today and continues to grow.

With her anorexia still under control more than two years after her therapy, Janice evaluated her treatment:

> Well, I still will judge myself too harshly and think myself beneath others at times, but I have a much higher regard for myself now. I am kinder to me, more loving to me, able to take a compliment and voice my opinion. One very important thing I learned and now notice with others is that if you take time for yourself, you are able to give more to others—be more loving and therefore more loveable. Positive does attract positive.

MOST EATING DISORDERS REQUIRE PROFESSIONAL ATTENTION

Dr. Louis K. Boswell points out that the chief nutritional problem of poor people in this country is obesity. He calls the situation here a matter of quality not quantity, and reveals causes for the problem found under hypnosis:[2]

> Under hypnosis, one of the most common self-images that overweight people struggle with is of feeling poor, poor in intelligence, poor in mate-

> rial and spiritual possessions, even though they may have all they need and want. Many of my patients who are successful in losing weight attribute their success to shedding a false belief that they are impoverished and poor. New attitudes and a success-oriented outlook on life help them develop better eating habits and a healthy body image.

Rarely are people able to recall, on a conscious level, the initial sensitizing event that causes their eating disorders. Under hypnosis, however, an analyst can examine occurrences in early life that cause people to consider food as more than simply fuel. When those sensitizing events are discovered and analyzed, the patient can let them go and accept the positive input, namely that food is only fuel. Only then can permanent weight control occur. People who ride the diet see-saw without changing their self-images have difficulty kicking their weight problem.

Past-life Regression in Treating a Ponce de Leon Syndrome

With permission from the *Medical Hypnoanalysis Journal*, I include here my article on treating an interesting case of the eating disorder bulimia.[3]

> Past-life regression is used by some therapists as a tool in treatment. It can be very effective as part of the regressive work in hypnoanalysis. In the example that follows, a past-life regression experience was the pivotal point that seemed to help this client through an impasse.
>
> Helga (fictitious name) appeared in my office two years ago with numerous complaints: depression, suicidal thoughts, low self-esteem, impending divorce, poor impulse control (she was beating her oldest son). She also reported a lack of control over her life, and that she was suffering from extreme guilt and bulimia. After I treated her with several psychotherapeutic approaches that I've learned over the last 15 years, including Transactional Analysis, Bodywork, Gestalt, Reparenting, etc., she managed to clear up some of her depression, raise her self-esteem, get out of an unhappy marriage, stop beating her child, and contain her suicidal impulses. However, the bulimia persisted.
>
> By highly confrontational group methods and warm, supportive psychodynamic individual treatment, she inched along, "making progress." However, she began regressing steadily. She began carrying around a stuffed animal she called "Blinky." "Blinky's" debut came after an intense session during which Helga began to understand her extreme dependence upon, and ambivalent feelings toward, her mother. Helga was 32 years old at this time. She had four children of her own. Helga herself is the youngest of three children. She grew up in a born-again fundamentalist religious environment and felt both psychologically and religiously conscripted to her family.

Bulimia has been called the emotional disorder of the 80's. Many hypotheses exist for its causes. Bulimia is a secret addiction that dominates the thoughts of the person (recent studies show that 95 percent of all bulimics are women). Bulimia undermines the patient's self-esteem and can endanger the person's life. Bulimia has also been called bulimarexia, the gorge-purge syndrome, bulimic anorexia and bulimic hyperemesis.

The excessive vomiting can cause death from cardiac arrest, kidney failure, and impaired metabolism due to electrolyte imbalance or severe dehydration, according to Lindsay Hall in *Understanding and Overcoming Bulimia.* Hall states further, "Other serious physical side effects include rotten teeth, digestive disorders, amenorrhea, malnourishment, anemia, infected glands, throat blisters, internal bleeding, hypoglycemia, and ruptured stomach or esophagus." These are only the physical possibilities.

Current psychotherapies for bulimia seem to focus on a behavior approach along with insight-oriented treatment. One of the key issues with bulimics is an avoidance of growing up. This may be reinforced by parents who unconsciously do not wish to let their children emancipate. In addition, the bulimic who has relied upon the approval of others to validate her self-worth may experience tremendous fear at having to trust inner resources in dealing with the world. These phenomena belong to a syndrome hypnoanalysts call the Ponce de Leon syndrome:[4] Helga was a classic example.

Since Helga began treatment with me, she has been receiving therapy based on several frames of reference. As a result of my induction to and subsequent residency in hypnoanalysis, Helga agreed to hypnoanalytic treatment.

From Helga's History

Q. What's the problem?

A. My problem, um, I guess you could say mood swings—a feeling of lifelessness, comatized. I don't know—feeling little in a big world—I'm scared about being normal.

Q. How long has this been a problem?

A. Three years—Actually it began way before—specifically when I was a kid and intensified when I was a teenager.

Q. What makes it better?

A. Sex—it snaps me out of it, snaps me into a different mind set.

Q. Traumatic incidents?

A. Being born (laughs).

Q. Describe your eating habits for me.

A. I try not to eat. Either I don't eat or I binge.

Q. Nervous habits?

A. I suck my pacifier.

Q. Describe your childhood to me.

A. It sucks! It was mediocre, middle, well, it was pretty ordinary: Father's an asshole, mother's a bitch—you don't break any rules, you just do what you're told.

To the question, "When you were born or your mother was carrying you was there any kind of problem?" she responded: "She didn't want me when she was carrying me." So, for an ISE, I would expect prebirth or birth. Her word-association test showed the following:

Fear . . . life

Life . . . death

Death . . . black

Hate . . . death

There must be . . . life after death

Live . . . die

Birth . . . death

All my life . . . nothing

The real problem . . . dying

Hypnosis . . . dying

Being normal is . . . dying

Most of all I want . . . to die

I resent . . . being born

Black . . . sex

It snaps me out of it . . . my kids

These responses seemed to indicate WZS (walking-zombie syndrome).[5] After her birth regression and a regression to three years of age, she did not release the extreme nature of her symptoms. However, she appeared to feel somewhat better and was interested in the origin of her feelings.

The real change took place after I explained to her (while she was in hypnosis) the dynamics of the Ponce de Leon syndrome and asking what happens after death. The dialogue follows:

Q. What happens after death?

A. I don't want to die.

Q. What happens after death?

A. You go to hell!

Q. Why?

A. For not being good, sinning.

Q. What's your first sin?

A. Being born.

Q. So, there's no way you can avoid it, is there?

A. No.

Q. Then what would a child do caught in this dilemma?

A. I don't know—probably feel dead.

Q. Yes, but there's one other thing a child might do and that's to not grow up, because if you don't grow up you don't have to die. Isn't that so?

A. YEAH!!! But how can I get out of it? I'm afraid.

Q. Suppose that you knew exactly what happens right after death. Would that help?

A. Yes.

Following that, I age-regressed Helga back to the life immediately preceding this lifetime. She told me she was an American Indian who was being burned for going against the tribal rules concerning sexual conduct. Helga described the excruciating pain of the fire. Tears flowed and she yelled out; finally a calm came over her face; the tears stopped. I asked her what happened. With disbelief in her voice, Helga said the pain was gone now and that she was above the body momentarily, drifting toward a light above.

I asked her about hell, Saint Peter, God in judge's robes and heaven. She replied negatively and reported meeting people (spirits) she had known who had died before her. "What are they doing?" I asked. She told me they were welcoming her. These people were happy to see her. "Do you feel peaceful now?" She said "yes."

Her trance demeanor never changed. The astonishment remained in her voice, and her face displayed the look of wonder.

Since Helga's attention span lasted only a few minutes, I decided to go on immediately. I told her to let go of everything she had experienced and blank her mind. "Now, on the count of three, you'll be at the time right before you entered your current body: one . . . two . . . three . . . where are you?"

Claiming that she had just entered the three-month-old fetus, she told how she already felt the conflict in her mother and already felt rejected and dead. At this point, I tied the elements together and instructed her to put an end to her fear of death, which she did willingly.

As a result of this past-life regression, Helga, who had displayed spiritual zombie tendencies throughout her history and who did grow up in a strict Christian fundamentalist home, was able to let go of her fear of dying, her fear of hell, and her fear of growing up. This was the turning point: She began focusing on having an adult life instead of acting out her Ponce de Leon fantasies, and even stopped carrying "Blinky." She wrote a story entitled, "Vanessa Grows Up." With Helga's permission, I'm recounting the first sentence. This sentence is indicative of the changes she made after this regression.

"One day it happened. Vanessa looked at herself in a full-length mirror and said, 'I love you; you're beautiful.'"

Helga was a fairly difficult case for me. Traditionally, she would have been classified as a borderline personality disorder, since she displayed many of the features associated with a diagnosis of borderline. Too often, when a therapist treats someone with these issues, the traditional bag of tricks is soon exhausted. The therapist experiences burn-out, with feelings of helplessness and worthlessness.

I was beginning to feel as if I were at the end of my rope with this case when, fortunately, I became a hypnoanalyst and, with these powerful techniques under my belt, was able to turn the case around.

Helga wanted to be married and have another child. She already had four children from two marriages. By the time she was getting ready to separate from her therapeutic relationship, she was experimenting with relationships. Not long after that, she met a man, married him and moved out of state. Recently, she visited Illinois with her newborn in tow.

SELF-HYPNOSIS AND VISUALIZATION HELP IN EATING DISORDERS

After taking a client's history, the routine I follow with weight-control patients includes completing a related word-association test, interpreting the patient's weight-related dream and regressing under hypnosis to locate the initial sensitizing event. After the patient recognizes the cause of inappropriate eating patterns and deals with that event, the remainder of the treatment is supportive in nature and emphasizes the deconditioning aspects of habitual behavior.

I suggest the following behavior for recovery:

- Set realistic short-term, intermediate, and long-term goals for body weight.
- Eat your first meal within one hour of waking.
- Eat small, well-balanced meals for lunch and dinner with no snacks between meals.
- Drink no alcoholic beverages when working on weight control.
- Practice self-hypnosis daily.
- Imagine yourself at the weight you want to be.
- Affirm your visualization with positive statements such as, "I look like I am __________ (sexy, thin, etc.)."
- Remember that the positive image you see of yourself is the one your subconscious will aim for.
- Get regular exercise.
- Continue to grow in self-love, developing an attitude of continuing maturity.

Key Concepts

- Obesity is a complex matter involving psychological, physiological, social, and physical components.
- Diets alone fail because they do not address the real problem.
- Exercise alone is neither efficient nor effective in reducing weight.
- An emotional attachment to food motivates people with obesity and eating disorders.
- Weight control needs to be attacked on three fronts:
  —Psychological/emotional issues
  —Eating habits
  —Activity levels
- Perceived threats to one of our survival prerequisites may be dealt with by overeating, resulting in obesity; by refusal to eat, resulting in anorexia; or by such behavior as bingeing and purging (bulimia), or other self-destructive actions.
- Unless the underlying negative suggestion or suggestions to the person's survival is removed, any attempts at dieting and food management will be counteracted by the survival mechanism.
- Through hypnoanalysis, persons not only can receive immediate symptomatic relief from life-threatening eating practices, but also can achieve a permanent resolution of the problem.

Growth Exercise

1. Keep a journal defining your relationship to food. Keep in mind the following questions:
   a. How do you know when it's time to eat?
   b. Do you eat when you're not hungry?
   c. How do you feel when eating breakfast? lunch? dinner? snacks?
2. Remember: Diets don't work. Die(t) is the message to your subconscious mind.

CHAPTER NINE

PHOBIAS: THE UNBEARABLE FEARFULNESS OF BEING

Worrying isn't necessarily
bad, but ruminating
over and over about what
awful thing can
happen is useless.

—*Ralph Waldo Emerson*

Men are not afraid of things,
but of how they view them.

—*Epictetus*

THE PLAGUE OF ANXIETY DISORDERS

Anxiety disorders, which include phobias and panic attacks, constitute the number one psychiatric problem in the United States. About 15 percent of the population is affected by at least one anxiety disorder; 11 percent takes anxiolytic drugs for up to 90 symptoms associated with anxiety disorders. About 6.5 million women and 3.5 million men suffer from tension that they are unable to deal with effectively. Arthur B. Hardy, M.D., publisher of the *Terrap Times*, estimates that about 13 million Americans suffer from some kind of phobia. By some estimates, as many as 8 million of these phobias are severe enough to have serious effects on their victims' mental health and their ability to function socially and vocationally. The Anxiety Disorders Association of America in Rockville, Maryland, estimates that as many as 24 million Americans —almost 1 in every 10—will suffer from some kind of phobia during their lifetimes. The number of phobics in the country rises to 100 million—about 40 percent of the population—if you classify as a phobia the most widespread fear of all: the fear of public speaking.

Some quick definitions:

- A **phobia** is an irrational fear or anxiety involving certain objects, persons, places, or situations.
- **Anxiety** is a low-grade, generalized fear.
- **Panic** is a sudden, unreasoning, hysterical fear.

I will give more detailed descriptions of these conditions later in the chapter. But for now, let's deal with the common denominator of all these conditions: fear.

FEAR CAN BE FRIEND OR FOE

Dr. Hardy, gives us this definition of fear:

> Fear is a reaction which warns us of danger. This reaction is intended to insure our survival. It is beyond our control. The fear reaction signals the body to run away and hide from danger. If you can't hide, or you are cornered, you will use the energy to fight your way out. The bodily feelings produced by this reaction are generally called "the symptoms of anxiety." [1]

Fear pumps up the nervous system, creating the impulse to fight or flee. The bodily symptoms of preparing to fight or flee include a rapid heartbeat, heavy breathing, tension, and warmth. These reactions are normal and can't be controlled. They are part of our nature. Throughout our history, human beings have needed to get pumped up to avoid dangerous animals, warriors, or natural disasters. Fortunately, for most of us, this is no longer the case. Many people, however, still experience this response, even when there is no real danger. These are people who suffer from irrational fears. Their bodies react as if survival threats were imminent, even though they may be quite safe. Consequently, stressful conditions result because of constant readiness to fight or flee.

Much unhappiness ensues from these conditions. Those who learn to control their reality (inner experience) largely determine their quality of life, which accounts for a functional definition of peace. Phobia sufferers cannot control their realities. Hence, they are very unhappy.

ANXIETY: SMALL-SCALE FEAR

Anxiety is a generalized, small-scale fear reaction indicating a possible danger. The danger frequently eludes the person, but the feelings are usually undeniable and uncomfortable.

Anxiety causes a dual reaction, both physiological and psychological. The symptoms are connected, impossible to separate. However, depending on some unknown vulnerability, some people will tend to experience more physical symptoms while others will experience more mental/emotional symptoms. A combination of symptoms is more likely.

Humans can experience two basic types of anxiety: exogenous and endogenous. Exogenous anxiety is the type most familiar to us. It's the type you experience when you can clearly identify the threat to your security or safety. When you're driving down the interstate and see a big semi closing in on your rear bumper, you experience exogenous anxiety. When your company is threatened by a hostile take-over and you perceive that your job is in jeopardy, you experience exogenous anxiety. The word "exogenous" means "originating externally." Your anxiety response is triggered by circumstances outside your body.

Endogenous anxiety stems from conditions within the person. Evidence indicates that it is a disease to which certain individuals are vulnerable. Endogenous anxiety attacks usually come without warning. The victim experiences anxiety without knowing why. Some of the symptoms are a racing heart, shortness of breath, dizziness, choking, or tingling.

It does no good to tell the victim of endogenous anxiety to relax, take a vacation and forget about the problem. That prescription might work for normal anxieties. But although the symptoms of endogenous anxiety may resemble those of normal anxiety, the two conditions are quite different.

The anxiety scale in Figure 9.1 shows the range of anxiety, from panic to butterflies in the stomach, along with the symptoms and effects at each step on the scale:

10	Panic: disoriented, spacy, detached, frantic, hysterical, numbness or weird sensations and feelings	AREA OF NON-FUNCTION
9	Dizziness, nausea, diarrhea, visual distortions, numbness, some hysterical sensations, concern for losing control	
8	Stiff neck, headache, feeling of doom	
7	Tight chest, hyperventilation	
6	Lump in throat, strong muscle tension	AREA OF DECREASED ABILITY TO FUNCTION
5	Dry mouth, feeling of need for escape	
4	Shaky legs, feel tremor	
3	Rapid or strong heartbeat, tremor, muscle tension	AREA OF CONTINUED ABILITY TO FUNCTION
2	Sweaty or clammy palms, warm all over	
1	Butterflies in stomach	

Figure 9.1
Reprinted with permission from Arthur B. Hardy, M.D., from page 2 of *Everything You Wanted to Know About Phobias But Had No One to Ask.* For more information, call **1-800-2-PHOBIA.**

PHOBIA: IRRATIONAL FEAR

Phobias are inordinate and irrational fears or severe anxiety reactions to certain situations, objects, or people that do not normally create fear in most people. Manuel D. Zane, M.D., and Harry Milt define a phobia as "a disorder in which the individual reacts with irrational dread and panic in a harmless situation, flees to rid himself of the unendurable sensations and feelings aroused in the situation, then henceforward, avoids it and similar situations, to avoid the anticipated recurrence of this extremely painful experience."[2]

The phobic reaction doesn't stem from some real threat. Rather, it is caused by an onslaught from the imagination. The phobic situation unleashes a frightening salvo of thoughts and images. The body starts pumping away as if these thoughts and images represented reality. If the victim were facing some real threat—an attacking dog, or a car approaching in the wrong lane—the mind could order a rational response. But since these are imaginary threats, the mind sees no way to deal with them. It, therefore, spurs the body on in an exaggerated response that can lead to panic.

The word phobia originates from the Greek word *phobos*, meaning fear. Individual phobias get their names by taking a Greek or Latin word for the triggering condition and combining it with the word "phobia." Thus, "phobophobia," describes the fear of fear that Franklin Roosevelt referred to in his first inaugural address, when he reassured the American people during the Great Depression that "the only thing we have to fear is fear itself."

The fear of loud noises and the fear of falling are the only two fears people are born with. All others are acquired or learned. Although phobia sufferers consciously recognize that the situation, object, or animal of which they are so frightened poses no threat to their lives or safety, they often will go to any lengths to avoid the fear-producing situation. It is then that phobophobia develops, causing people to alter their life-styles and relationships in dramatic and crippling ways.

Phobophobia is real to many people. It frequently follows the onset of another phobia, so the sufferer fears the fear itself as much as the situation or object that provokes the fearful response. With some phobias, the symptoms progressively intensify until phobophobia prevents some patients even from leaving their houses or—in extreme cases—their rooms.

Phobias are not new. Hippocrates described a phobic (a person with a phobia) some 2,400 years ago:

> He would not go near a precipice, or over a bridge or beside even the shallowest ditch, and yet he could walk in the ditch itself.
>
> When he used to begin drinking, the girl flute-player would frighten him; as soon as he heard the first note of the flute at a banquet, he would be beset by terror. He used to say he could scarcely contain himself when night fell; but during the day (when people were about him) he would hear this instrument without feeling any emotion.

From historical and literary references, we learn that phobias have existed throughout the world and throughout history. The Anxiety Disorders Association of America in Rockville, Maryland, estimates that 1 American in 10 suffers from phobias at some time during their lives. They live in New York City and in Pogosa Springs, Colorado. They live in Miami Beach and in Bluefield, West Virginia. They include illiterates and Ph.Ds, Protestants and Catholics, Jews and Muslims. They're found among mechanics, college professors, artists, garbage collectors, and corporate CEOs.

Phobic reactions can be frightening experiences. As Zane and Milt note:

> A situation sensed by the phobic person to constitute a threat—even though no actual danger is perceived or recognized—sets off an automatic reaction of the entire system, which in turn generates a chain of frightening thoughts, images and secondary bodily reactions. Instantaneously, the mind's attention and the body's reactions are captured to the exclusion, for the time being, of all else. The response is automatic, comprehensive and consuming.[3]

PANIC BREEDS PHOBIAS

Phobias frequently grow out of panic disorders. Panic, remember, is a sudden, unreasoning, hysterical fear. Panic attacks are episodes of irrational terror mainly accompanied by symptoms of sweating, heart palpitations, chest discomfort, faintness, trembling, hot or cold flashes, feelings of unreality, or fear of losing control or dying or of going crazy. Many panic sufferers believe they are having heart attacks and seek emergency-room help. Panic attacks usually begin during times of general psychological distress. As a result, a phobia related to the place, situation, or person may develop in response to the panic.

The person experiencing a panic attack develops a feeling of total disaster. Emotions seem driven to the wall, with no avenue of escape. The situation seems unbearable and unendurable, and the victim often feels that the only recourse is to faint, go berserk, or die.

THE LONG LIST OF PHOBIAS

In the play *The Merchant of Venice*, Shakespeare wrote of "some, that are mad if they behold a cat." Anticipating Sigmund Freud by centuries, Shakespeare was describing a phobia. It is through the writings of Freud, the father of psychology, that the most common phobias are known—acrophobia (fear of heights), agoraphobia (fear of public places), claustrophobia (fear of closed places), xenophobia (fear of strangers), homophobia (fear of gays), zoophobia (fear of animals), even—get this—triskaidekaphobia (fear of the number 13).

If you want to be left to yourself at a party, memorize these phobias and spring them on your friends:

Aurorophobia—fear of the northern lights
Barophobia—fear of gravity
Blennophobia—fear of slime
Cryophobia—fear of cold
Cyclophobia—fear of bicycles
Diabetrophobia—fear of diabetes
Dikephobia—fear of justice
Gallophobia—fear of French things
Geniophobia—fear of chins
Kopophobia—fear of exhaustion
Leukophobia—fear of the color white
Methyphobia—fear of alcoholic beverages
Mnemophobia—fear of memories
Patriophobia—fear of heredity
Peladophobia—fear of bald people
Panophobia—fear of everything
Phasmophobia—fear of ghosts
Photoaugiophobia—fear of glaring lights
Scabiophobia—fear of scabies
Tuberculophobia—fear of tuberculosis
Uranophobia—fear of heaven

You can research additional names yourself. There are about 180 of them defined. With a little imagination, you can add to the list. Just take any place, object, sound, smell, color, or condition that could possibly excite fear, find its English, Latin, or Greek name, and put it in front of the word "phobia."

Regardless of the number of phobias, there's only one phobic feeling reaction: FEAR. It results in decreased functioning, avoidance, and unhappiness.

THE CAUSE IS THE KEY

"The triple allergenic theory indicates that a person is sensitized or set up for a particular reaction to certain stimuli," writes therapist Nicholas Cooper-Lewter about the initial sensitizing event (ISE) or root of a phobia.

> From this point on the person is a potential time bomb of symptoms and problems. Symptom-producing events lurk in the person's life. Symptom intensifiers strengthen the potential strangle hold a person's disease may bring.[4]

When dealing with phobias, a trained hypnoanalyst will be able to uncover the subconscious origin of a problem. Subsequent sessions will undo this subconscious knot and free a patient to live a healthier, more productive life.

The misunderstandings about phobias and the ways professionals of various disciplines try to classify them are rampant. Classifying phobias so that we have 180 or 18,000 does not solve the real problem. What matters is how the client has accepted the fearful suggestion and how we are going to deal with it through hypnoanalysis. Although a phobia may be totally reshaping an individual's life, the fear itself is a magnification of the root problem. We need to be searching for the initial suggestion generating the fear—the ISE.

Most phobias are deep seated. They tend to remain embedded in the subconscious and continue to cripple individuals for months or years if they are not removed through treatment. Phobias and panic attacks don't usually go away by themselves. However, some cases lie dormant for periods. I have had extensive training and several years of experience, both as a psychotherapist and as a hypnoanalyst, and have found that the most effective way of dealing with phobias is to conduct word-association tests and age regressions. The word-association tests link ostensibly unrelated words through subconscious recognition, leading to the target age for the ISE. Once removed, the other stages of treatment must follow (the eight R's referred to in the Introduction).

I agree with Lewter that, like other emotional problems, phobias can always be traced back to an initial sensitizing event. Dr. Louis K. Boswell, whom I've referred to several times already, described the cause and recommended treatment of phobias this way:

> An event sufficiently dangerous to the individual may give rise to a state of anxiety in that individual's mind and continue to influence the personality for a long period of time. Threatening events superimposed on this initial sensitizing event will serve to magnify the intensity of the original anxiety. As each threat produces even greater anxiety, the fear for survival takes on an aura of reality. . . . We must pay particular attention to those which produced a real threat to the patient's survival. . . . We must analyze each problem in the light of this ultimate fear—physical or emotional death.[5] (I would add to this the spiritual component as well.)

THE THREE PHOBIA TYPES

Phobias are generally classified into three groups: simple, social, and agoraphobia. People with simple phobias are afraid of singular, identifiable objects or conditions. Fear of heights, water, particular animals and insects characterize simple phobias.

Social phobias involve public situations. People with such phobias may experience anxiety while attending parties, eating in restaurants, speaking before groups, or in other situations in which they are conscious of being observed by other people. The anxiety manifests itself in the form of physical symptoms such as trembling hands, blushing, perspiring, dizziness, weakness in the limbs, palpitations, and hyperventilation. When the victim experiences these effects, the usual response is to flee from the situation and to avoid such situations in the future.

FEAR OF PUBLIC SPEAKING

Fear of public speaking is a social phobia. As noted earlier, 40 percent of Americans are victims of this fear, which is also known as performance anxiety. It can be a severe handicap for those whose jobs require them to communicate with groups.

I've worked with many people who would rather walk on hot coals than speak in public. I can attest to the self-imposed limitations to career, self-confidence and personal satisfaction this fear causes. But does this fear qualify as a phobia?

Burton J. Rubin, author of the *Stage Fright Handbook*, tells us:

> By all accounts, more people are afraid of public speaking than anything else. . . . [Performance anxiety] consistently outpolls the fear of disease, loss of a loved one and even fear of death itself in fear studies. Perhaps this is not so surprising at all when you consider that communication, speaking and conveying our thoughts, is the primary way by which we interact with others. Every time we express ourselves in one manner or another, we reveal ourselves and put our egoes, our self-images on the line.

Further, Rubin says:

> In contrast to fear, a phobia is an irrational fear. A phobia is also a fear of fear. I believe that anxiety, discomfort caused by sympathetic nervous-system reasons in, or in contemplation of, a public-speaking environment qualifies under either definition.[6]

I agree. The main issue in fear of public speaking is that many people can simply avoid the opportunity, whereas other phobic reactions cannot be avoided by scheduling or by refraining from volunteering.

But for some people, public speaking is a career requirement. A man named Ken came to me for help after hearing one of my lectures on the subconscious mind. He was embarking on a new career that required him to speak weekly to a different group of professionals. He told me:

> Every time I think of getting in front of a group of people, I freak out. I get scared to death. Not only that, but when I actually do have to start talking, I get diarrhea and sweaty palms, and my armpits get so wet I'm afraid that I'll embarrass myself in front of the group.

Ken was an intelligent, good-looking man in his thirties. I asked him when his problem began.

"I had it in high school so bad that I would skip school on those days when I was supposed to speak," he told me.

"How did you get through college?" I asked.

"Well, I used a lot of courage and would avoid taking classes where I had to get in front of the class."

"What makes it better?"

"Not having to do it?"

"What will you be able to do once this is cured?"

"Enjoy giving speeches."

During the word-association test, Ken told me his problem began at the age of nine. Actually, the number nine appeared in his history several times. The subconscious always sends clues to the astute analyst.

During his eighth session, I regressed him back to a time in his ninth year. Relying on the assumption that the subconscious always knows what the problem is, I told him: "On the count of three, we're going back in time to a scene, memory, or feeling that's directly related to your problem." I counted to three and snapped my fingers.

"What's happening?" I asked.

Ken answered: "I'm in the gym. They're all looking at me and I can't talk. I'm crying. I feel terrible, embarrassed. I hate myself." He sobbed. "What's wrong with my voice?"

The scene took place at a Cub Scout Jamboree when Ken was nine years old. He was the master of ceremonies and was to introduce the next act. When he got in front of the packed gym, he froze and couldn't speak. A teacher finally rescued him from the situation.

Once he realized the impact of this childhood scene, he was able to let go of the fear that paralyzed him in his adult life. It was the fear of repeating the situation that took place when he was a third grader—the fear of looking foolish again in front of an audience. Ken resolved his phobia and now speaks regularly. He even looks forward to it.

Direct Suggestion May Remove the Fear

Hypnoanalysis revealed the key to Ken's problem. Mary Kullman, a colleague of mine, solved another speech-fright problem through direct suggestion. She was approached by Sally, a 38-year-old sales executive, who was experiencing anxiety as she contemplated a speech she was to give in her Dale Carnegie course. Sally told Mary:

> My chest gets tight when I start to talk; my voice sounds like it is somebody else's voice. I panic, and when I notice that my voice sounds funny and shaky, I need to take a breath but I can't. When you're up there you can't do it. I get all quivery and my hands shake.

Mary asked how long she had experienced the problem.

"Probably since high school," she said. "I honestly think it started in grade school. In gym, the teacher would pick on little fat kids, and I was a little fat kid."

Sally had the same teacher for three years.

"When I'm standing," she said, "I still feel like a little fat kid."

Mary resolved this case in two sessions by giving Sally direct suggestions. She helped the patient realize that she was not a little fat kid anymore. By strengthening her self-image and building her confidence, Mary enabled Sally to make her Dale Carnegie presentation. Mary gave her a subconscious trigger mechanism to counteract the symptoms whenever she began to experience performance anxiety. Sally called back and said everything went fine.

No Magic Formula

There is no magic formula for overcoming the anxiety associated with public speaking, but confident speakers turn their nervousness to an advantage. They take their anxiety as a sign that they are emotionally ready for the speech.

For most people, though, the nervousness compounds the problem. They are convinced that the audience is waiting for them to make a mistake and will ridicule them for every little miscue.

In fact, the audience is not waiting for them to make mistakes. Most audiences don't even notice the speaker's nervousness, and if they detect mistakes, they are prone to overlook them.

You can go a long way toward overcoming your fear of the podium by revising your attitude toward the speech. The people who feel the greatest anxiety about speaking in public are those who view the speech as a performance. Those who are most comfortable with public speaking are those who see it as an exercise in communicating.

Observes Michael T. Motley, Ph.D., professor and chair of the Department of Rhetoric and Communication at the University of California, Davis:

> Excessive anxiety is especially common among people who view speeches as performances, in which they must satisfy an audience of critics who will carefully evaluate gestures, language and everything else they do. Though they can't describe precisely what these critics expect, people with a performance orientation assume that formal, artificial behavior is somehow better than the way they usually talk.[7]

Giving a performance requires that you be an actor or an actress. Few of us are blessed with that talent. So it's better to be yourself. That doesn't require acting. And, what many have discovered is that being yourself is more than enough!

Motley has a technique he uses to help his speech students "be themselves." Here's how he describes it:

> As the speaker approaches the podium, I dismiss the audience temporarily and begin a 'one-way conversation' with the speaker. I tell him or her to forget about giving a speech and simply talk spontaneously to me, using the speech-outline notes as a guide. In this situation, most people

> feel rather silly orating, so they start to speak conversationally, using natural language, inflections and gestures. I ask the speaker to maintain this conversational style while the audience gradually returns, a few people at a time.[8]

Speakers are usually able to maintain the conversational quality before the full audience. When they don't, notes Motley, "the transition from talk to speech is invariably identified later by the audience as the point when effectiveness began to decrease and by the speaker as the point when anxiety began to increase."[9]

Here are some of Motley's tips on overcoming the fear of speaking:

- Decide on your specific objectives first. Before you think about anything else, know one or two major points you want to communicate. Then, plan the best way to get them across.
- Put yourself in your audience's place. Recognize how you and most of the audience differ in attitudes, interests, and familiarity with what you are talking about. Then, speak to them on their terms, in their language.
- Don't memorize and don't read. Except for a few carefully chosen gems—memorable phrases or examples you know will work well—be as spontaneous as possible. Don't rehearse to the point that you find yourself saying things exactly the same way each time. Use brief notes to keep yourself organized.
- Speak to one person at a time. Looking at and talking to individuals in the audience helps keep you natural. It feels foolish orating at one person. Speak to that person as long as it is mutually comfortable, usually up to 15 seconds.
- Try not to think about your hands and facial expressions. Instead, concentrate on what you want to get across and let your nonverbal communication take care of itself. Conscious attention to gestures leads to inhibition and awkwardness.
- Take it slow and easy. People in an audience have a tremendous job of information processing to do. They need your help. Slow down, pause, and guide the audience through your talk by delineating major and minor points carefully. Remember that your objective is to help the audience understand what you are saying, not to present your information in record time.

- Speak the way you talk. Speak as you do in casual conversation with someone you respect. Expecting perfection is unrealistic and only leads to tension. The audience is interested in your speech, not your speaking.
- Ask for advice and criticism. For most people, careful organization and a conversational style add up to a good speech. A few speakers, however, have idiosyncrasies that distract an audience. Solicit frank criticism from someone you trust, focusing on what might have prevented you from accomplishing your objectives. Usually, people can correct problems themselves once they are aware of them. If you don't feel you can, take a course in public speaking or see a speech consultant.[10]

Rubin contributes these tips:

- Stay in the present; don't worry about what's ahead with all the "what ifs" and "how do I knows?" You can stay in the present by concentrating on some object in the here and now, such as a table, chair, sofa, or lectern.
- Concentrate on speaking with emphasis. If you're concentrating on the words you're going to stress and the way you're going to interpret your material, you won't have the mental capacity to think ahead and worry about the "what ifs."
- Don't panic when you "go blank." Actually, you haven't gone blank at all. The information and the words you want are there in your brain. You just aren't directing your mental energies toward finding them. Instead, you're caught up in the thought that "I am going to go blank," or "I've just gone blank." Clear the mind of these thoughts and concentrate your mental efforts on remembering the information you need. Often, speakers go blank when they try to keep too much information in their heads at once. Take it one thought at a time, and don't worry about the next three thoughts.
- Accept the fact that you have stage fright, and concentrate on doing the things you're supposed to do. The more that you accept the fact that you have stage fright, the less panicky you will get.[11]

Toastmasters International is an excellent organization for those who want to develop their public-speaking and leadership skills. Toastmasters gives you a chance to speak before a friendly audience of peers in a relaxed and pleasant setting. Chapters are found in communities throughout the United States. Notices of meetings are often published in local newspapers and are posted on public library bulletin boards. You can write to the organization at Toastmasters World Headquarters, 2200 North Grand Avenue, P.O. Box 10400, Santa Ana, California 92711.

AN UNUSUAL PHOBIA

Fear of public speaking is the most widespread of public phobias. Less common, but also less avoidable, is the fear of urination. I haven't had a patient who complained of the fear, but the issue has arisen in the case histories of several male patients.

Usually, the problem surfaces only when other men are present, and the sufferer approaches a urinal with other men standing beside him. As the person feels his urine begin to flow, he actually feels more anxiety and fear of not going, or of dripping on his pants. (Actually, an analysis of a urination phobia would be interesting to do.)

SOCIAL PHOBIAS STRIKE WHILE YOU'RE YOUNG

We often find that social phobics were shy and timid during childhood. Adolescence finds them lonely and socially isolated. They usually experience their first attacks between the ages of 15 and 30. After that, their phobias may strike again and again for many years.

Social phobics are extremely self-conscious and sensitive to the ways they are perceived by others. Social phobias often are rooted in disturbing childhood experiences.

AGORAPHOBIA

Agoraphobia takes its name from the Greek word *agora*, meaning marketplace or a place of assembly. A German psychologist, Dr. G. Westphal, gave it the name after he had dealt with three patients who experienced terror associated with various places in which they happened to be. It could be a workplace, a certain street, a certain building, or a certain square.

Westphal described the phobia as "the impossibility of walking through certain streets or places or the possibility of doing so only with resultant dread or anxiety."

Some have since characterized agoraphobia as a fear of open spaces, but that is misleading. The anxiety can strike indoors or outdoors. A victim may experience it while standing in a grocery checkout line or waiting at an airport baggage claim. When a person experiences such an attack, the typical reaction is to avoid such a setting in the future. The anxiety spreads to other locales, and soon the victim may feel safe and comfortable only at home or in the immediate neighborhood of home. Often, a person suffering from agoraphobia finds it impossible to function away from home or outside the presence of a trusted friend or relative.

Alan Goldstein, Ph.D., a psychologist and director of the Agoraphobia and Anxiety Treatment Center in Philadelphia, tells us that agoraphobia often stems from childhood conditions. Agoraphobics frequently come from homes in which the parents were either overprotective or too distant. Often, one or both parents was an alcoholic or an agoraphobic, or suffered from some illness or other condition that required the child to shoulder too much responsibility. Many agoraphobics, as children, felt threatened by separation from their parents, or actually experienced the separation. Some experienced sexual abuse. Observed Goldstein:

> Because agoraphobics don't have the power, as children, to change their distressing circumstances, they learn to adapt by habitually denying their family problems and the feelings they have about them. Then, as adults, instead of dealing head-on with conflicts in their relationships, they become chronic avoiders, never complaining for fear of rocking the boat.[12]

Depression is a frequent companion of social phobias and of agoraphobia. Everyone experiences mild depression once in a while. It's the feeling of dejection you feel when things aren't going right for you. You've had a run-in with the boss, you've just lost a big sale you'd been counting on, your marriage or your romance has hit a few bumps, or a friend has let you down in some way. In most lives, there are enough positive experiences to offset these letdowns, and the blues will pack up and leave after a short stay.

But sometimes, the downers in life are so severe and the reaction is so deep and intense that depression moves in for a long visit. Such long-lived depression often accompanies the loss of a child, a spouse, a sibling, or some other person who is close to the victim. Divorce or the breakup of a long-standing romantic relationship can also trigger depression. So can phobias that cripple one's ability to function normally in situations involving other people.

Fortunately, most people have the resources to recover from the pitfalls of life. For those who cannot recover on their own, hypnotherapy offers a means of uncovering the hidden basis of the depression. In the case of phobias, hypnotherapy can help the patient to expunge from the subconscious the factors that bring on the phobia. When the phobia is gone, the patient can deal with the depression.

A phobia is very real and not something that's just "in your head." Phobias often strike intelligent, hard-working people and haunt their lives like waking nightmares. Some phobias will appear without warning and disappear as quickly, but those that last for more than a couple of months hold tenaciously to their victims unless treatment is sought.

Peanuts cartoonist Charles Schulz is a well-known sufferer of agoraphobia. Rheta Grimsley Johnson, author of a recent Schulz biography, credits the artist's chronic condition with his creativity:

> Most things are sad to him sooner or later. Everything becomes a source of depression. . . . His loneliness is not the kind most of us feel when a loved one goes (or passes) away. It is baseless and unrelenting and must be dealt with as a basic bodily function—daily, unremarkably, constantly. And the sad, conspicuous irony is that without this wellspring of grief, there most certainly would not be the humor, the piercingly clear look at human foibles and insecurities, the Charlie Brownness of life that have made the cartoonist rich, famous, and funny.[13]

Schulz, according to Johnson, is among the agoraphobia victims who suffer panic attacks when faced with strange settings, long-distance travel and some public places—hotel lobbies, for instance. She quotes him: "Just the mention of a hotel makes me turn cold. When I'm in a hotel room alone, I worry about getting so depressed I might jump out of a window."[14]

A young woman's letter that appeared recently in the Ann Landers advice column described the typical onset of anxiety attacks and received an empathetic reply from the columnist.

> Dear Ann Landers:
>
> I am a 24-year-old female who needs your help. Lately I have had what I believe are anxiety attacks. The first one occurred while I was driving home about a month ago. I managed to make it, but was really frightened because I had no idea what was happening to me. My sister told me to sit down and take several deep breaths. She put a cool cloth on my face and I did feel better, but let me describe the feeling.
>
> Your body shakes and your heart beats like a trip-hammer. There is shortness of breath, you feel lightheaded as if you are going to faint, and you think for sure you are having a heart attack. It really is scary.

> I went to a doctor, who prescribed a drug. I had heard that some of these drugs are addictive and can change your personality.
>
> I don't want to take drugs, Ann. I want to fight this thing on my own. Please tell me what to do.
>
> Hopeful in Detroit

Ann's reply:

> Dear Detroit:
>
> You are courageous to want to fight this on your own, but it may not be possible.
>
> I hope you will seek out a mental health professional who specializes in phobias and related anxiety disorders. For additional information, contact the Phobia Society of America, P.O. Box 42514, Washington, DC 20015.
>
> You are not alone. Millions of others have experienced anxiety attacks, and with the proper help they have gotten them under control. You can too. Good luck.[15]

Ann's advice is good. The fear of panic attacks often moves untreated victims to the next step of severity: phobic avoidance—avoiding the situations, people, and places where panic attacks have occurred. Finally, full agoraphobia may result, and suffering individuals will fear being away from what they consider "safe" persons, places, or situations. They will alter relationships and behavior patterns in dramatic and crippling ways. They will redesign their activities and life-styles to avoid fear-producing situations. Depression often accompanies agoraphobia, as does seeking relief through alcohol or drugs.

Joy Considered Suicide

Joy came to my office complaining:

> Well, I have panic attacks. I've had them for a long time. I feel like everything's unreal. I get tense and shake. That started happening in eighth grade. I started smoking pot; I thought I was going crazy through high school. They went away during college. After I graduated, they got real bad. It's gotten worse now that I'm home.

I wondered what she would like to do that these problems stopped her from doing. Her answer:

> Lead a normal life; to feel like I don't have to worry. I hate being alone. I have a strange feeling that I'm two people. I feel worthless and half the time I don't feel like living. I don't know the meaning of life and I feel useless.

During her analysis, I regressed her several times. I took her back to the womb, to the time of birth, and to traumatic events and accidents that might have been the ISE. However, the panic attacks returned, although Joy was improving in all areas of her life. She met a man, got married, left her parents' home, and began law school. Joy reported greater self-esteem and more zest for life. But those panic attacks were stubborn, and I knew I was missing something.

Joy grew up with an alcoholic father and possessed the qualities of an adult child of an alcoholic. That fact, though, didn't explain the troublesome attacks. The answer surfaced in relation to Joy's mother and how Joy could get her needs met.

During panic attacks, said Joy, "My mother comforts me." During her upbringing, Joy learned that to get her needs met within her family she had to get very needy. Once she understood what she gained from continuing her panic, she learned healthier ways to take care of herself.

This was an interesting and challenging case because I couldn't solve it just by finding and bringing to consciousness the initial sensitizing event and the symptom-producing event. I had to uncover and analyze the secondary gain—the conditioning factors in her relationship that supported her intense fear.[16]

Joy credited hypnoanalysis with saving her life. She wrote:

> I probably would have committed suicide if I hadn't sought help. This experience has made me alive again. . . . I no longer feel dead and worthless. Although I still have problems, I don't face them with the intense fear and dread that I once did. [Hypnoanalysis has been] the most beneficial experience in all my life.

Phobias and panic disorders are curable with professional treatment involving client and family education, the restructuring of negative thinking, and support for confronting the feared situation while resolving any conflicts uncovered. Sometimes, medication is necessary. The important thing is to identify the problem and get professional help to face the fear.

MOST OF US AVOID *SOMETHING*

Fear is a natural and normal feeling, as are the other feelings humans experience, such as anger, sadness, and happiness, in varying degrees. There are about 100 words describing feeling. I've only included the four basic ones.

Phobics, however, seem to have their fear stimulated more easily and more intensely than other people do. Phobics experience the feelings others do; it's just that their fear predominates.

The following poem puts the condition in perspective. Written by Don Mesuda, Jr., it appeared in a newsletter of The Phobia Society of America:

My Phobic Friend

My phobic friend is a special person,
One who cares without rehearsin'
Some can't drive or be alone,
But would rather prefer to stay at home.
Others feel funny in public places,
And get very nervous when meeting new faces.
My phobic friend needs special attention
Because new situations cause much apprehension.
Sometimes it's hard to understand,
But imagine living in a foreign land.
Or having a constant panic attack
With thoughts of lions at your back.
My phobic friends need people to confide in
So they won't need their shells to hide in.
They've missed some parties and summer vacations,
But are thankful for their family's patience.
For without support, the phobic is alone,
Their dearest resource is the telephone.
They have learned to face their fears,
And look forward to ending years of tears.
After weeks of practice they finally see
How wonderful life is when you're Phobia-free!

THE FEAR OF FLYING

I think this poem is clever, pointedly sincere, and timely. I would add just two lines, after "apprehension" in line 8:

When it comes to boarding a plane to fly,
My dear phobic friend would rather die.

A great many of my clients come seeking help with aviaphobia (fear of flying). The Boeing Aircraft Corporation published a recent survey in which it claimed that more than 25 million Americans are afraid to fly. If nearly 20 percent of the American population is afraid to fly, aviaphobia is more common than even I thought it was.

Since the media have been flapping for several years about near misses and mid-air collisions and the like, any air incident only aids and abets the panic felt by fearful flyers. The reality of flying is that it's safer, statistically, than driving a car.

People with aviaphobia have vivid imaginations and do not need the media to produce horrific fantasies in which they see themselves on a crashing plane, suffering all the lethal consequences in dramatic color. Media coverage tends only to reinforce the fear of flying and the attitude that "I'll never fly again. It's too dangerous."

Removing the Fear

For one middle-aged lawyer, fear of flying had its roots in a difficult birth experience. He came to me complaining of anxiety each time he had to fly or use an elevator. Interestingly, it wasn't the flight or the elevator ride that frightened him; he was quite comfortable during flight. It was the contemplation of flight that caused him to break into a sweat. That suggested to me that the problem originated in the womb.

I regressed him back to the womb and he told me:

> I feel pushing, squeezing; it's tight . . . a floating sensation . . . pulling . . . stuck, trapped. . . . I don't know what to expect. I am being pulled through. It's wet, scary. They put me down.

At that point, I had him identify his fear in the here and now. He pinpointed it at the moment he was getting onto an elevator or into an airplane. I asked him to leave it in the past, and he did. I deconditioned his subconscious mind, relieving it of that fear of moving into closed, tight objects. Some time later, he told me he was still flying and enjoying it very much. His case was a complete success!

Tips for Aviaphobics

Since flying is so common in our present life-style, and the fear of flying creeps up in most of us at one time or another, I thought I would include some specific suggestions that may be helpful in dealing with aviaphobia:

- Do NOT watch television programs, news coverage, or survivor interviews after a plane crash. There is little benefit from these publicized accounts.
- Do NOT take air accidents personally as "Just my luck, I've got a flight coming up and wouldn't you know it, there's a crash."
- Do NOT engage in superstitious or magical thinking. Air accidents are not omens, portents, or harbingers of the future. Nobody has the psychic wherewithal to cause an air crash. Air crashes do not happen in numerical sequences such as three in a row; nor do they take place more frequently on Friday the 13th or during a full moon or when Mercury is in retrograde.
- Keep in mind that all air accidents are thoroughly investigated by the government and airlines and, after reviewing the findings, changes are policed by regulatory agencies for improving safety and performance.
- Remember that all near misses are not catastrophes narrowly prevented. A near miss can mean planes are still miles apart.
- Keep in mind that not everyone stops flying after a crash. Only those predisposed to phobias do. Others just get nervous for a time.
- Telling yourself something like "I only have a number of safe flights in me" is useless and induces more fear.
- Don't watch disaster films such as *Airport* or the like. They just feed negative fantasies.
- If you're phobic, get help.

WHAT PHOBIAS HAVE IN COMMON

In my practice, I treat many people who are suffering from phobias. It doesn't matter what the phobia is. It could be anything from fear of water to fear of crowds. Basically, they're all the same in that they come from the same source—the subconscious mind. Some belief within the subconscious is causing this fear.

Through hypnoanalysis, I communicate with the subconscious mind. With the client's help, we are able to identify the source of fear, analyze it, resolve it, decondition it, and remove it.

Remember, you have nothing to fear but fear itself. Conquering fear is only a matter of going within yourself and pulling out the root cause of your phobia. After that is done, you'll truly understand the last line in "My Phobic Friend," "How wonderful life is when you're Phobia-free."

Key Concepts

- Phobias are irrational fears or severe anxiety reactions to certain situations, objects, or animals that do not normally create fear in people.
- The fear of loud noises and the fear of falling are the only two fears people have from birth.
- Most phobias are deep seated, and their victims need help from hypnoanalysts trained to conduct word-association tests and age regressions, or from a comparably trained professional.
- Like other emotional problems, phobias can always be traced back to an initial sensitizing event. There was a time before the fear existed.
- Phobia sufferers will redesign their activities and life-styles and will alter relationships and behavior patterns to avoid fear-producing situations.
- Depression and relief-seeking, along with self-destructive behaviors such as controlled-substance abuse, often accompany phobias.

Growth Exercise

Refer to the chart on page 142. What areas of your life correspond to the various levels of anxiety?

____

____

____

If none, be happy!

CHAPTER TEN

CODEPENDENCY: THE BASIC HORROR OF IDENTITY

Ever since people first existed, they have been doing all the
things we label "codependent." They have worried themselves
sick about other people. They have tried to help in ways
that didn't help. They have said yes when they meant no.
They have tried to make other people see things their way.
They have bent over backward to avoid hurting people's
feelings and, in doing so, have hurt themselves. . . .
They have believed lies and then felt betrayed. . . .
They have worn sackcloth because they
didn't believe they deserved silk.[1]

—*Melody Beattie*

Creative minds always have been known
to survive any kind of bad training.

—*Anna Freud*

A NATION OF CODEPENDENTS

What is a codependent? The term is usually applied to family members of alcoholics and drug addicts, but it can apply to anyone who has had to live in a dysfunctional family or with an abusive person. Those who must deal continually with dysfunctional persons adjust their own behavior to compensate. They use this compensating behavior to deal with the addicted or dysfunctional person.

Notes Donald Brennan in the *The Recovery Press*:

> Many psychologists, such as Claudia Black and John Bradshaw, believe that anyone who has been involved, especially in childhood, with chemically dependent persons in long-term intimate relationships has been pathologically affected by those relationships. The consequent mental disorder is called "codependence," and it is a widespread malady in any society where substance abuse is prevalent. Therapist Sharon Wegscheider-Cruse estimates that as many as 96 percent of Americans could be affected.
>
> Ann Wilson Schaef, in her book *When Society Becomes an Addict*, maintains that U.S. society itself is an addictive system, and that in our time the American people are collectively codependent, with relatively few in recovery. The vast majority are caught in the throes of this progressive disease, and expend tremendous energy in their efforts to survive the symptoms. It is a majority out of touch with feelings, entrenched in denial, and caught up in role-playing, disordered thinking, enabling, and all manner of debilitating, dysfunctional and addictive patterns of behavior. According to Schaef, codependence permeates not only our families but our institutions and their bureaucracies, including businesses, schools and government.[2]

Humans compensate for many things in many ways. If you begin to develop a near-sighted condition, you unconsciously begin to squint when peering at distant objects. By narrowing the opening through which your eyes peer, you sharpen the distant image somewhat. Of course, the permanent remedy is eyeglasses or contact lenses. Once you have the proper lenses, you don't need to squint any more. But you may still do it out of habit. You are still trying to control your eye focus by squinting, even though you no longer need to do so.

When one member of a family develops a significant dysfunction, it upsets the balance in the family arrangement. Everybody's role changes somewhat. Everyone has to adjust.

WHEN FAMILY BALANCE IS UPSET

The family unit has been compared to a hanging mobile. The mobile is in delicate balance. If you change the position or weight of one of the hanging units, you disrupt the balance of the entire mobile.

If Dad is an alcoholic, a workaholic, or a golfaholic, he will not exert his full weight on the family mobile. If Mom is a drug addict, a clubaholic, or a shopaholic, she too will throw the mobile out of balance. If the addict is Dad, perhaps Mom steps in, becoming a self-sacrificing martyr as she assumes the roles of both parents.

Or maybe the oldest son assumes the burdens his father won't assume. In such a case, he becomes a family "hero," sacrificing his childhood for the good of the entire unit. The oldest daughter may similarly assume the responsibilities of a dysfunctional mother—or of both parents. The child has become trapped in a behavior mode dictated by the parent's dependency, and thus becomes a codependent. By shielding dependent persons from the consequences of their actions, codependents enable them to continue and, even deepen, their dependencies.

Codependents, therefore, are enablers. An enabler, according to Angelyn Miller, "is one who prevents growth and learning in others by assuming their responsibilities. An enabler promotes weakness in others by protecting them from the consequences of their unproductive behavior."[3]

Observes Jennifer P. Schneider, M.D., author of *Back from Betrayal,* in her foreword to Miller's *The Enabler:*

> Enablers, as adults, often continue to consider themselves innocent victims who are making the best of a bad situation. Surrounded by crises, they "pull the family through" time and again. They are often seen as heroes by their friends.

Miller cites the alcoholic as "the classic example of the dependent who needs the support of others to maintain dependent patterns." She explains:

> Alcoholics who find a mate who will accommodate their behavior can spend a lifetime without changing. They have someone strong and capable they can depend upon to hold things together, cover for them, and protect them from the consequences of alcoholism. Dependents believe themselves to be victims of an uncaring world, when actually they are victims of an overprotective one.[4]

The codependent wife tells the kids Daddy is sick when he's actually drunk. She calls the boss to tell him Joe is sick and can't come to work when Joe's ailment is a hangover. When makeup won't hide the shiner he gave her last night, she tells friends she ran into a door instead of into the fist of a drunken spouse. The codependent wife is sick and needs help as much as her alcoholic husband.

Codependents feel powerless to stop the addictive behavior or correct the personality vulnerability that feeds their codependency. They seek, instead, to control the behavior that results from the disorders. They assume responsibility for others' behavior and welfare. This self-sacrificing behavior becomes embedded in the subconscious and distorts the codependent's relationship with the rest of the world.

Children who grow up in a dysfunctional home will find it difficult to function in normal surroundings. Their subconscious minds have adapted their behavior patterns to the abnormal environment, and when they take those patterns into normal settings, the patterns don't mesh.

Codependents grow up believing that their mission in life is to be at the service of others. But fulfilling that desire does not lead to a warm feeling of contentment. It frequently leads to unhappiness. They often feel victimized.

Codependency is a much broader problem than drug or alcohol addiction. Codependents, says Schneider, "learned their unhealthy behavior as victims of a painful or difficult childhood." Frequently, as the product of a dysfunctional family, their nurturing was inadequate. These codependents-in-training learned how to cope with a difficult family life by becoming rescuers and caretakers, thereby confusing being loved with the feeling of being needed. Schneider characterizes adult enablers as "volunteers rather than victims."[5]

THE MAKING OF A CODEPENDENT

Marty, a 50-year-old optometrist, came to my office seeking weight loss. After taking his history, I learned that Marty is a codependent, but his codependence didn't grow out of an alcohol or drug environment. It grew out of a dysfunctional home in which Marty had to assume parental responsibilities at an early age.

"I'm mother and father to the world," he later told me. He didn't identify codependence as a problem; he simply felt helpless and too fat.

Marty's father, Luther, was a man of lower-than-average IQ, though Marty's grandparents had never acknowledged it and had never sought special training for their son. Marty's mother, Margie, was a bright woman who had grown up in a poor family with no educational tradition. Her face was disfigured by a large birthmark. As a teenager, Margie had no suitors except for Luther, who was a ninth-grade dropout. Margie herself quit school to marry him.

Marty was the oldest child, and as younger brothers and sisters came along, he had increasing responsibility for their nurturing. Both his parents had to work the graveyard shift at a local factory—from midnight to 8 A.M. From the age of nine onward, Marty was left in charge of his younger siblings while the parents were at work. He also had to baby-sit them during the afternoons following school so that the parents could get their sleep.

Throughout high school, Marty could not engage in extracurricular activities because he had to be home with the younger kids. He could have no social life because that would conflict with his child-care duties.

On top of filling in for both parents as the caretaker for his younger siblings, Marty became a partner in the denial of his father's mental handicap. Marty became adept at shielding his younger siblings from his father's temper. He became adept at modeling his own behavior so as to avoid rousing his father's anger. He became a codependent from an early age.

When Marty grew up, he joined the military, then attended college on the GI Bill. Though he became a successful optometrist, he did not outgrow his codependence. He married a woman with emotional problems and became a buffer between her and his children. He also tried to keep her problems hidden from their friends.

Marty grew up absorbed in the needs of others to the neglect of his own. He spent the early part of his life living in reaction to his father's moods and behavior. He spent his adult life responding to the needs of his disturbed spouse. Consequently, he resorted to overeating as a way of dealing with his own needs, which he couldn't identify until several months of therapy had elapsed.

So, having an alcoholic or a drug addict in the family is not a prerequisite for codependency. One can develop codependency in dealing with anyone close who has emotional or behavioral problems.

In her book, *Codependent No More*, Melody Beattie produced this definition of codependency:

> A codependent person is one who has let another person's behavior affect him or her, and who is obsessed with controlling that person's behavior.[6]

Miller's definition is similar:

> . . . (P)eople who need and use others to maintain nonproductive and self-defeating behaviors. It is a parasitic relationship—the **dependent** needing (or wanting) someone to take over his or her responsibility to society, and the **enabler** needing (or wanting) to take over another's responsibility in order to bolster his or her own sagging self-image.[7]

Often those who seem to thrive on problems are feeling dead inside and therefore, need the drama and excitement that problems create in order to know (subconsciously) that they are alive. Codependents need dependents and vice versa.

Beattie lists these characteristics of a codependent:[8]

- **The need to take care of others:** Codependents feel responsible for other people. They anticipate other people's needs and wonder why other people don't anticipate theirs. If you need something that they can provide, codependents feel obligated to provide it. If codependents need something and you give it to them, they feel guilty for accepting it. But after they've done so much for others, they often feel angry, victimized, unappreciated, and abused. Codependents lead sad lives, never realizing they are volunteers in their codependency.

- **Low self-esteem:** Codependents live in abnormal environments, but they pretend that everything is normal. They blame themselves for everything but get angry, defensive, self-righteous, and indignant when others blame them or criticize them. They reject compliments but get depressed when they're not complimented. They feel guilty about having fun just to be having fun. In fact, guilt is their constant companion.

- **Tendency to repress feelings:** Codependents are afraid that if they acknowledge their thoughts and feelings they will be overcome by guilt.

- **Worrying:** Codependents focus all their energy on other people and their problems but never find the solutions.

- **Controlling and being controlled:** Because the behavior of other people has brought them sorrow, codependents are afraid to let other people be themselves. To exercise control, they may feign helplessness, or they may try to use guilt to influence the behavior of others.

- **Denying there's a problem:** Codependents don't like to face problems head-on. They prefer to wish them away—push them out of their consciousness and pretend they don't exist. They have trouble acknowledging how bad things are. They believe lies—even the lies they tell themselves. Thinking magically, very often they exhibit symptoms of the Ponce de Leon syndrome.

- **Depending on others for happiness:** Codependents look for happiness outside themselves and attach themselves to the people or things they think can bring happiness. Their quest for love and approval often draws them to people with problems. But often, the people they're drawn to are incapable of loving. Codependents eventually feel trapped in relationships that don't work and stay with them long after healthy persons would have walked away.
- **Difficulty in communicating:** Codependents tend to communicate indirectly. If they don't say what they mean, it's often because they don't consciously know what they mean. Their true feelings are submerged somewhere in their subconscious. They ask for what they want or need indirectly, through sighing or pouting or other nonverbal methods of communicating.
- **Inability to draw the line:** Codependents don't know how to set boundaries. They'll draw lines in the sand, then keep blurring the lines. Eventually, they will put up with what they said they'd never put up with, do things they said they would never do. They let others hurt them—repeatedly—then wonder why they hurt so bad. All the while, they feel victimized.
- **Lack of trust:** Codependents don't trust themselves, their feelings, their decisions, or most people. Yet, they try to trust untrustworthy people. They think God has abandoned them and often lose faith and trust in God.
- **Anger and fear of anger:** Codependents are afraid to express anger because they're afraid they'll make other people angry. They get depressed and cry a lot. They may overeat. Eventually, their repressed anger explodes in a "get-even" act of hostility, or in a violent outburst of temper.
- **Problems in the bedroom:** Codependents take their controlling behavior into their bedrooms. They may be more concerned with pleasing their partners than with pleasing themselves. Sex becomes another act of self-sacrifice.

THINGS MAY GET WORSE

If a codependent fails to get help, the condition can have serious repercussions. Depression and lethargy are among the by-products of codependency. Codependents may become withdrawn and isolated. Feeling trapped in their relationships, they may begin planning ways out. Sometimes the way out is suicide. They may become violent and seriously ill, emotionally, mentally, or physically. They may overeat, undereat, or abuse alcohol and other drugs.

Codependency is largely an identity problem. John Bradshaw, in his book *Homecoming, Reclaiming and Championing Your Inner Child*, defines codependence as "a disease characterized by a loss of identity."[9]

John Scott, Sr., a colleague and hypnoanalyst from Memphis, Tennessee, characterizes codependency very well in this script for an audio tape, which I play to codependent clients while they are in hypnosis:[10]

Who Am I?

> One might say, "Who am I?" Codependents are people who do not know what their lives are all about. They seem to be floating aimlessly along without specific goals. They do not have much ambition, which in turn indicates that they do not have very much energy either. So as they float through life without aims, goals and ambitions, they are like matchsticks tossed about on the water.
>
> The inner self, which is called the ego, is weak and brittle. This is indicated sometimes by the person's saying that he or she feels shaky inside. This shaky or insecure feeling inside causes a person also to be a little bit afraid about the future. Codependents are not sure what the future holds for them. A person in this position does not have an inner sense of cohesion or connectedness. There is no sense of power. Another way that some people look at it is that the inner self is scattered or fragmented. They feel that their lives are in bits and pieces.
>
> Some codependents describe themselves in this way:
>
> "I am unwanted."
>
> "I am unlovable."
>
> Others feel that when they were born they were not planned, so they have no purpose and feel that they are some kind of a mistake. They will frequently conclude that there is no reason for their existence into the future. And frequently they reveal that they are unable to cope with life.

> Some . . . turn to vices such as drugs, alcohol, smoking and obesity. . . . they [frequently] have an intense fear of rejection. Many times they feel that their behavior is more childlike than adult. They lack the security and the strength that an adult has. Some people have recurrent depression and grief. Some also feel that they have lost contact with God and therefore they have a very empty feeling about themselves, spiritually and emotionally.

Scott says the problem is often traceable to prebirth experiences. He notes:

> There is a kind of extra-sensory perception in the communication between the mother and the unborn child. It is as if in the last three months before birth the child in the womb is like a mind reader. And it reads the mind of the mother. Severe events in the daily life of the mother can send messages to the unborn child by means of the hormones that are secreted by the mother and in turn flow into the unborn child.
>
> The strong emotions of the mother, which are manifested by fear, anger, hatred or pain, frequently will influence the unborn child. Before the child is born it is very sensitive to these emotions. . . .
>
> Sometimes the mother's feelings are that the pregnancy is unplanned and unwanted and has no purpose; that it is a mistake. And if the mother has these feelings strongly, week in and week out throughout the pregnancy, there is a chance that the unborn child will absorb those feelings and believe these feelings are its own before it is ever born. If the mother has feelings of bitterness and resentment and disappointment, these strong emotions also produce feelings in the unborn child that are similar. . . . So a person can have an identity problem due to the events that happened before that person was born.

The attitude of the father affects the unborn child indirectly through the mother. If the father neglects or abuses the mother, her attitude is affected and she passes this on to the child.

Identity problems may also arise from conditions in early childhood. As Scott tells us:

> Before a child is five years old, it is in a perpetual state of hypnosis, which simply means that the child is highly sensitive and picks up quickly on all that goes on around him or her. The events and the feelings that have a strong impression on the child influence that child's feelings about itself. And so, if it is born into a home where it is unwanted and unloved or (what's worse) where it is abused; where there is rejection on the part of mother or father or both, then that too works away on the new infant, and puts within its mind a feeling of not being wanted; of being rejected; of having no cause to be alive. If the child was born prematurely or if it was born too late or if it had an unusual birth situation, this too can influence the child. It doesn't always, mind you, but sometimes it does.

When the child feels unwanted or like an intruder into the world, notes Scott, it may respond through some form of self-destructive behavior. The child may even become accident-prone or illness-prone, which means that it is subject to many illnesses all of the time. In some cases, even more serious illnesses such as cancer and diabetes are likely to develop.

"In most all of these situations," Scott observes, "the person is unable to love." This is the one trait that is common to all people who have identity problems. They do not have the capacity to love, especially to love themselves. Even if they start to enter into a love relationship or they have a relationship that looks like it might be love, it doesn't last. Something happens to those relationships that keeps them from getting deeper.[11]

Such people are also unable to enter into a loving, trusting relationship with God. They may belong to a religion and profess belief in God, but they understand neither God nor religion. They do not feel deeply spiritual in their relationship with God, so they are unable to develop a deep love for God, for themselves, for someone else of the same sex, or for someone of the opposite sex. Usually these people have a confused relationship with their parents.

Often, it takes time for codependents to volunteer the information that identifies them as codependents because they submerge themselves so completely in the task of caring for and controlling others that who they are has long ago slipped out of sight. Because they feel that they exist for others, they overlook self-care.

A codependent may have worked hard throughout life to become successful in a career. Having achieved success, the ordinary person would feel perfectly justified and comfortable in indulging in some kind of reward: a trip around the world, an expensive new car, or a nice sailboat. Ordinary people can do that for themselves and enjoy the fruits of their labors.

But codependents can't be carefree. If they spend that kind of money on themselves, they will be haunted by feelings of guilt, and they won't be able to enjoy the things their labors have purchased. Therefore, many codependents who are outwardly successful, with every apparent reason for happiness, nevertheless feel hollow and incomplete on the inside. They may isolate themselves, then suffer through depression and loneliness. Not knowing who they are, they overlook the possibilities in themselves. They ignore the opportunities for personal growth and fulfillment.

He Had a Spirit!

Arthur, a codependent 40-year-old male, showed up for treatment after being involved in various forms of therapy groups and modalities for nearly 20 years. Arthur said:

> My problem . . . is that I can't stand to be myself. Secondly, I feel stuck in my career. I want to change, but I don't know what to do with myself.

I asked what he wanted from me.

> I want the freedom to be myself without having to cling to somebody. Also, I want to make a change in my living and working situation.

Art grew up with an alcoholic father and a very controlling codependent mother. He expressed anger and frustration over having worked on his problems since the early 1970s and still feeling the way he described.

After doing his word-association tests, Art brought in a dream he had. This is it:

> I wonder if I have a spirit in me that doesn't belong there. Sometimes I feel like my head is full, as if there's an extra consciousness along for the ride.

His word-association test showed the classical signs of the identity problem:

RYAN: Complete a sentence beginning with the word "who."
ART: Who am I?
RYAN: Unwanted . . .
ART: Me.
RYAN: They really wanted . . .
ART: Somebody else.

But what really turned this case around was the regression connected to his dream. Art regressed to a scene in which he was in the crib. His mother had just lost his month-old sister, who died of a problem heart. Art described in vivid detail, with tears, the terror of being beaten by a desperately depressed mother. He was helpless and he writhed with pain as each blow reached him. His spirit died during those beatings. He lost the connection and love of his mother.

Once he understood this, relived the experience, and realized his mother had acted crazy, we brought his spirit back to life. With the help of much reinforcement he was able to love himself again. It took a while, but he solved his problem, left a dead-end job, married, and moved out of state.

CHILDREN ARE VULNERABLE

Children are particularly vulnerable to codependency. They easily fall into the trap of mistaking codependency for love. This mistaken perception can follow them into adulthood and can lead them into marriages or romantic relationships that are built on codependency. Art's relationship to women replicated the one he had with his mother. He tried to please and became overly concerned with her needs.

Children of addicted parents may express their codependency in a number of ways. They may do it by overachieving—pushing to be the best in school or in sports. The object is to counteract the shame of the addiction by giving the family something to be proud of.

They may try to be entertaining, seeking to relieve the tension at home by being amusing and never taking anything seriously. It's no accident that the best comedians often come from dysfunctional homes.

They may cope by withdrawing from the family, spending a lot of time alone or with friends. Or they may choose rebellion—acting outrageously in an effort to distract attention from the family's core problem. This was Art's strategy, which he had resolved before engaging in hypnoanalysis.

Art's spirit was dead. He couldn't keep the greatest commandment in the law, according to Jesus, recorded in Matthew 22: 36–40, "Love God with your whole heart, soul and mind. And the second is the same as the first, love thy neighbor as thyself."

Art is on his way to loving himself.

Child abuse and neglect have a profound negative effect on a child. When children get abused at an early age, healing requires recognizing the feelings and memory, rehabilitating thoughts and behavior, reeducation (in Art's case, this meant accepting he was a child of God first and of his earthly parents second), and reinforcement and repetition of the positive suggestions. Lastly, healing requires taking responsibility for feelings, thoughts, and patterns, regardless of where they began.

Addicted to Religion

John Bradshaw's father was an alcoholic, and John became the family "hero" after his father abdicated his responsibility. Bradshaw became a superachiever in the Catholic school he attended, then decided to study for the priesthood. Now an author and lecturer on family problems, Bradshaw contends that religion can become addictive when you completely surrender your thinking and creative powers to a set of unyielding beliefs.[12]

Bradshaw identifies religious addicts as those people who are absorbed in religious activities to the exclusion of family, friends, and all secular interests. When a parent becomes a religious addict, the addiction affects the rest of the family much as any other addiction would.

"It's not uncommon in a family where there's religious addiction, where the parent is super responsible, to have the kids become underresponsible or underachievers," Bradshaw told a group at the Center for Recovering Families.[13]

When one member of a family gets out of balance, the rest adapt by assuming different roles. "The second you have to play a role," Bradshaw contends, "you no longer can be yourself. You no longer can be real. You start playing the role, and every one of these roles has prescribed emotions that go with it. . . . Your very choices are determined by the role. . . . A false self arises. . . . Once you get into these roles and they get ingrained, you think that's who you are. You think that's your essence. You think that's your identity. The fact is that you don't have any identity. All you have is a role."[14]

Adopting the role comes as a result of families being out of balance. In hypnoanalysis, we very often find that the balance was not there in the beginning, and by identifying the codependent's ISE, we can speed up recovery.

Shame Is at the Core

Bradshaw identifies the core problem as shame. The person who experiences shame feels flawed as a human being. Shame, in fact, is identified with the genesis of human flaws. It was shame that Adam and Eve felt when they were driven from Eden, no longer the flawless human creatures God had placed in the garden.

The Garden of Eden story takes on added significance when codependents realize that Adam and Eve ate from the Tree of Knowledge, which was reserved for God only. The result was judgment. After eating, they learned the difference between right and wrong, which was reserved for God only. The consequence of original sin is judgment. Judging one's self and others is part and parcel of shame. By stopping and relieving subconscious judgment, codependents can realize who they are.

Who Am I, Really?

Incorporating shame is a gradual and complex operation. Art's began with his physical abuse. Marty's began with the relationship to his parents. Others frequently report a womb experience as the onset of their shame. Resolving this problem is commonly done through recovery groups along with hypnoanalysis.

The person who feels flawed also feels hopeless. What do you do with flawed items? You cast them aside and look for one that's perfect.

"Codependency," says Bradshaw, "is a way of institutionalizing shame." "It's a way I can always feel good about myself because I'm always helping others."[15]

In reality, codependents do not feel good about themselves. They struggle through life dealing with their shame, trying to shield the objects of their codependency from shame, taking responsibility for others, but neglecting their own primary responsibilities: the responsibilities for themselves.

Once recovery has progressed and the codependent realizes and feels that he is a child of God first and a child of his parents second, the battle is half over.

GUILT, LONELINESS, AND DEPRESSION

Guilt, loneliness, and depression are the handmaidens of codependency. Guilt sticks to codependents. They have assumed enormous responsibility—the responsibility for the welfare of the family or for the behavior of their dependent partners—and when they are unable to control things for the better, they blame themselves.

Guilt can be a healthy force when it warns you in advance of a wrong course, or when it reminds you after the fact that what you did was not in your best interests and should not be done again. Healthy guilt is a gut feeling.

It becomes unhealthy when it takes charge of your mind and actions long after the need for remorse has passed. Unhealthy guilt is obsessive and needlessly repetitive.

The codependent's guilt is based on the need to be perfect and on the feeling of being guilty of existing. Codependents are extremely tolerant of imperfection in others but can't tolerate it in themselves. Therefore, when they fall short of perfection—as all humans do—they are unforgiving of themselves.

Writes Joan Borysenko, Ph.D., author, psychologist, and cell biologist: "When you overcome the tyranny of black-and-white thinking and accept the range of grays that makes us human, you'll begin to let go of unhealthy guilt."[16]

Borysenko has some other healthy advice that applies to codependents: "Quit people-pleasing, and be true to your own feelings. . . . Instead of repressing anger to appear virtuous and kind, express your feelings in an unhurtful way. Instead of doing things you don't want to do in an effort to win others' approval, stop being a martyr and learn to say no when it's appropriate."[17]

Codependency breeds loneliness. The codependent feels trapped in a one-sided relationship that provides no emotional nourishment. This spiritual famine is the essence of loneliness.

Codependents are lonely because they are unable to share themselves with others. They are unable to share themselves because they have no identities of their own. Their identities are lost in the identities of the people they are trying to control or please.

As Bradshaw writes:

> The wounded inner child contaminates intimacy in relationships because he has no sense of his authentic self. The greatest wound a child can receive is the rejection of his authentic self. When a parent cannot affirm his child's feelings, needs and desires, he rejects that child's authentic self. Then a false self must be set up.[18]

As one patient remarked to James F. Masterson, adjunct clinical professor of psychiatry at The New York Hospital Cornell Medical Center: "I'm not doing what I want, because my ideas—about how I work, how I think, how I dress—and even my hobbies and how I relate to men are filtered through the perception of what *others* want. I'm good at perceiving what pleases other people and giving them what they want, but I feel trapped, like I'm suffocating inside my skin."[19]

Codependents are afraid to allow themselves to become close to others because they are afraid of being engulfed on the one hand and abandoned on the other. To break this cycle of loneliness, the codependent must first recognize the problem, then develop more constructive ways to relate to people and life. Codependents must, almost literally, become new persons, developing interests and friendships on their own, apart from their partners in codependency. Hypnoanalysis, with its unique capacity to speak directly to the subconscious and go straight to the initial sensitizing event, can reduce considerably the time frame for the individuation process.

Guilt and loneliness, of course, produce depression. Depression has many causes—some genetic, some psychological, and some environmental.

Difficult relationships often support depression. A person may be drawn into a difficult relationship by psychological-codependent "needs," and this completes the cycle of depression.

Depressed people are persistently sad and anxious. They feel hopeless and pessimistic. Nothing ever turns out right, and nothing ever will. They feel guilty, worthless, and helpless. They have no interest in pleasures, hobbies, and activities they once enjoyed. They feel tired, listless, and apathetic. They sometimes think of death or suicide, and in extreme cases will attempt suicide. They have trouble concentrating and remembering things. They also have trouble making decisions. They are plagued by headaches, digestive disorders, and chronic pain.

In its pamphlet, *Plain Talk about Depression*, the National Institute of Mental Health, Office of Scientific Information, suggests these methods of dealing with depression:[20]

- Do not set yourself difficult goals or take on a great deal of responsibility.
- Break large tasks into small ones, set some priorities, and do what you can as you can.
- Do not expect too much from yourself too soon, for this will only increase feelings of failure.
- Try to be with other people; it is usually better than being alone.
- Participate in activities that may make you feel better.
- Try mild exercise, going to a movie or ballgame, or participating in religious or social activities.
- Don't overdo it or get upset if your mood is not greatly improved right away. Feeling better takes time.
- Do not make major life decisions, such as changing jobs or getting married or divorced, without consulting others who know you well and who have a more objective view of your situation. In any case, it is advisable to postpone important decisions until your depression has lifted.
- Do not expect to snap out of your depression. People rarely do. Help yourself as much as you can, and do not blame yourself for not being up to par.

There are a number of short-term pick-me-up techniques for pulling oneself out of blue moods. They may not solve the basic problem, but they may help get you up for that special occasion when you can't afford to be down.

First, figure out what's eating you. Often, when you sit down and think about it, you can pinpoint some event in the recent past that is out of your conscious mind but keeps bugging you from its subconscious retreat. Maybe it was a bit of criticism you didn't think you deserved, or some action on the part of a friend that you interpreted as a snub. It may be the weather, or simply loneliness.

By pinpointing the triggering event, you can decide on an appropriate action. It may be that you need only to be told, "I'm okay, even if the boss did criticize the punctuation in that report I submitted. I liked its substance, and that's what counts."

Exercise can help a bad mood. It can physically release pent-up feelings of anxiety. It can restore a sense of control over events. It also causes your brain to produce more endorphins, which are natural antidepressants.

You can use mental visualization—self-hypnosis—to replace negative thoughts with positive ones. Remember a happy period in your life and dwell on it. Or think of things that have made you laugh.

For women, shopping may be a surefire pick-me-up. Shopping makes you feel that you're taking care of yourself. For the codependent, shopping also reinforces the idea that you're an individual with the ability to make decisions on your own.

Reading a book or talking with a close friend will let you take a break from problems. But don't choose a book or a friend that will reinforce your depression.

Taking a drive or a walk, or spending some time in a natural setting, may give you the change of scenery you need. If your mood is associated with a particular room or office, get out of it for a while.

You can go anywhere you want in your imagination. Try planning an imaginary vacation—to Tahiti, to Monaco, or to Acapulco. Drop by your friendly travel agency and pick up some brochures. If you really want some vivid images, get a travel video.

If all else fails, throw a punch—at a pillow, a punching bag, or some other object that won't feel pain, won't strike back, won't be destroyed, and won't hurt you. You might try buying an inflatable clown that bounces back up when you hit it.

The point is that you have needs apart from the needs of your partner. Indulge those needs. Recognize that you're imperfect, too, and since you share that trait with more than 5 billion other human creatures, you don't have to feel guilty about it. Discover yourself, make friends with yourself—your inner child—and start treating yourself with the same kind of concern you show to others. Take yourself on a picnic, to the zoo, or on some other activity you enjoyed as a child.

SIX STEPS TO RECOVERY

Addictions, of course, can be cured. Recovery from codependency is also possible. Human Services, Inc., of Dallas, Texas, lists these six steps toward recovery:[21]

1. **Being honest.** Admit that your partner really is addicted to a substance or a behavior, and that both of your lives are being controlled by this addiction.

2. **Detachment.** Give up trying to rescue the addicted partner, to solve his or her problems, make him or her happy, or save him or her from the consequences of his or her addictive behavior. *This isn't within your control.*

3. **Putting yourself first.** Take care of your own needs. Plan activities and set goals for yourself that are not contingent on your addicted partner's moods or actions. *Only the addict can solve his or her problems; only you can make yourself happy.*

4. **Getting help.** Reach out to friends, relatives, or a therapist who can help you sort out your feelings and begin living for yourself. Without help, your codependency will get worse.

5. **Talking.** Recognize your own needs and feelings, especially the anger you may feel about the control the addiction has had over your life. Then tell your partner—without apologies—what you want.

6. **Being patient.** Understand that you won't solve your problems all at once, so don't try. Instead, take one step at a time and feel proud of your strength and courage.

The Alcoholics Anonymous Twelve-Step Program has been a useful model in helping people recover from codependency. As one codependent put it:

> When I began using a Twelve-Step Program, I heard a lot of talk about people using behavior to control others. They all seemed to know what this controlling behavior was, and they all seemed to agree there was

> something wrong with it. At first I didn't understand. When I finally understood, I got mad. I felt accused of doing something awful. It made me angry. I had been taught to seem powerless, had learned ways to appease my craving for love, attention and recognition in indirect ways because it wasn't acceptable to want those things, much less ask openly for them. But I was now being told it was my own sick controlling behavior that made others miserable and kept me from feeling close to them. Something inside me screamed, "Not fair! Not fair!"[22]

THE NEED TO CONTROL

Codependents have trouble recognizing that their unconscious need to be in control is compulsive. They don't know they have such a need, they don't know how to get rid of it, and they are surprised when others point it out.

But controlling others is rarely necessary. Others don't need our control. Rather, it's the codependent who has the need to control. That need springs from our subconscious and it is actually destructive. It keeps us from feeling and from facing reality.

How do you know when you're using controlling behavior? There are a number of signposts.

One is **tension**. If you're doing the controlling, you feel nervous because you're trying to manipulate someone into doing something to please you or not doing something that displeases you.

Another signpost is **blaming**. You point to someone else as the cause of your unhappiness. You try to make the other person feel guilty. When you do that, you're conceding to someone else the right to determine how you feel.

Urgency is another signpost. You're desperately trying to prevent something from happening, or you have this overpowering need to make something happen. That's a signal that you're trying to control.

The final signpost is **refusal to feel**. This shows up constantly in the codependents I treat. To be a codependent requires that you discount, deny, or ignore your own feelings and the feelings of others. Codependents don't want to know their own feelings or the feelings of others. This sometimes makes it difficult to determine the initial sensitizing event for a codependent person due to codependents' capacity to ignore their feelings and deny their problems. However, with the support of a group, and the eight R's of hypnoanalysis (Relaxation, Realization, Reeducation, Rehabilitation, Reassurance, Repetition, Reinforcement, and Responsibility), the ISE eventually emerges. (See the Introduction for more about the eight R's.)

The treatment plan for codependence has three guiding principles:

1. The cause is in the past. There have been experiences, events, and people, or the lack of these, over which the patient has had no control. These have left a hangover or ghost from the past, which has caused current problems.

2. No blame. We are not here to blame or point the finger at anybody. We are attempting to understand the past and its effect on your subconscious mind.

3. Working together. We work together so that understanding emerges gradually. We can't do everything at once. The pieces will fit together. We are headed in the right direction.

HOW TO LET GO

Since codependency is an instinctive response, it springs from the subconscious. That's what makes hypnoanalysis an effective means of uncovering the ISE and freeing the subconscious mind of the memories and attitudes that result in codependent behavior.

Codependents present the hypnoanalyst with a challenge, however. If hypnoanalysis is to be successful, the patient must have a trusting relationship with the hypnoanalyst. Yet, codependents have conditioned themselves to expect the worst from everyone. They're never sure of what others will do if they let down their guards. It becomes doubly important, then, for the hypnoanalyst to establish a relationship of trust with the patient. The patient must be shown how to turn loose the need to control.

How can this be done? The Hazelden Foundation, in its pamphlet, *Letting Go of the Need to Control*, gives several suggestions:[23]

1. Look for behavior patterns. Because the need to control is instinctive, it resurfaces time and again. Learn to recognize these instinctive reactions and you'll soon recognize your controlling *modus operandi.*

2. Make up your mind that you will trust your own feelings and perceptions. When you decide to believe in yourself, your self-esteem will rise.

3. Identify alternatives. Look at the way things are going now. If nothing changes, what real choices do you have? What are the probable consequences of each choice? You can try to get others to change by communicating with them indirectly—through hints, pouting, withdrawing, and other actions. You can wait until things are different. Or you can look for other choices that lie outside your habitual way of doing things.

4. Check out assumptions. Low self-esteem causes you to imagine the worst. You act as though what you've imagined is true, and your imagination becomes a self-fulfilling prophecy. But often your worst fears are groundless, especially when it comes to the way other people regard you. You need to ask more about what others really think and feel. When you take the trouble to check out assumptions, you are in a position to act on the basis of facts not fears.

5. Decide what you really need and start looking for it. Take a needs inventory at work and at home, with friends and family. Be candid. You deserve support in your efforts, and you must learn to trust those near you to provide the support. By learning to trust, you build self-esteem and you gain the strength to take risks. That strength will enable you to let go of your codependency and to recapture yourself for yourself.

The Twelve-Step Program has been an effective route to recovery for alcoholics and other substance abusers. It can also help codependents to recover. To follow the Twelve-Step Program, codependents must:[24]

1. Admit that they are powerless over the factor that brought on their codependency.

2. Come to believe that a power greater than themselves can restore them to sanity.

3. Make a decision to turn their will and their lives over to the care of God, as they understand him. (In my groups, and in hypnoanalysis, I work with God. God equals Love only.)

4. Make a searching and fearless moral inventory of themselves.

5. Admit to God, themselves, and to another human being the exact nature of their wrongs.

6. Become entirely ready to have God remove all these defects of character.

7. Humbly ask Him to remove their shortcomings.

8. Make a list of all persons they have harmed, and become willing to make amends to them all.

9. Make direct amends to such people wherever possible, except when to do so would injure them or others.

10. Continue to take personal inventory, and when they are wrong, promptly admit it.

11. Seek through prayer and meditation to improve their conscious contact with God, as they understand him, praying only for knowledge of His will for them and the power to carry that out.

12. Having had a spiritual awakening as a result of those steps, try to carry this message to others, and to practice these principles in all their affairs.

These general steps, while developed specifically for Alcoholics Anonymous, are useful for codependents as well. The codependent who follows these steps need not be in a relationship with a substance abuser. It could be anyone who was reared in a dysfunctional family.

As Angelyn Miller observed, the families of codependents "need a chance to get out from under the enabling of their caretaker, and their enabler needs to be relieved of the burdens."[25]

A good prayer for all codependents—one that can be used as a self-hypnosis suggestion—is this:

> God grant me the serenity to accept the things I cannot change, the courage to change the things I can, and the wisdom to know the difference.

Key Concepts

- A codependent is a person who has allowed another person's behavior to affect him or her and who is obsessed with controlling that person's behavior.
- The codependent's partner may be a person who is addicted to alcohol, drugs, or religion.
- When one member of a family develops an addiction or another type of dysfunctional behavior, the rest of the family members assume roles to compensate for the dysfunctional member.
- Codependents submerge their own identities while trying to control the behavior of others. They try to shield the objects of their codependencies from the consequences of their actions. They try to assume responsibility for the actions and welfare of others.
- Codependents are marked by a need to take care of others, low self-esteem, a tendency to repress feelings, a tendency toward excessive worry, a need to control and be controlled, denial that there is a problem, dependence on others for happiness, difficulty in communicating, inability to set boundaries, lack of trust, anger and fear of anger, and problems in sexual relations.
- Codependence breeds loneliness, guilt, and depression. Depression may breed codependence, and a cyclical pattern results.
- Codependence is an instinctive response; hence, the key to overcoming it lies in uncovering subconscious motivation.
- Hypnoanalysis can help by uncovering the ISE through age regression. This requires the building of trust between patient and analyst.
- The steps toward recovery are honesty; detachment; putting oneself first; getting help from friends, relatives or a therapist; and talking openly with your partner.
- To free oneself of the need to control, one should look for the behavior patterns through which one attempts to control, determine to trust one's own feelings and perceptions, identify alternative ways of coping with problems, check out assumptions to make certain that

choices are based upon facts instead of fears, and decide what one really needs and start looking for it.

Growth Exercise

1. Ask yourself whether you identify with the codependents described in this chapter. Be honest.
2. Analyze what are you doing to help yourself.
3. Read books by John Bradshaw or Melodie Beattie.
4. If you are depressed, seek professional help immediately, especially if you're suicidal.
5. List your own unproductive, self-destructive behaviors. Decide which ones you want to change.
6. Intuitively, give a percentage of the time you are living for others—from 0 to 100 percent. Do it now, without thinking. ________________.
7. Intuitively, what percentage of the time are you assuming responsibilities for others? ____________
8. Intuitively, what percentage of the time do you seek love from:
   God?________________.
   Others?______________.
   Self?________________.

- -

If the answer to Question 6 is over 15 percent, you need help. If your answer to Question 7 is anything above 0 percent, except for children, you need help. On Question 8, the mature score is God 33 1/3 percent, others 33 1/3 percent, and self 33 1/3 percent.

Nobody is perfect—remember that. However, mature people need to spread their need for love among the three sources.

- -

9. Consider this quote:

> The need to belong to something larger than ourselves underlies many of these pursuits. We long to feel a vital part of some community of others, to have the security that comes through belonging to something larger than ourselves. It is through identification that ultimately we know rootedness.[26]

   What do you think?

CHAPTER ELEVEN

WINNING IS MIND OVER MUSCLE; IF YOU DON'T MIND, THEN MUSCLE DOESN'T MATTER

It is not enough
to fight. It is the
spirit which we bring to the
fight that decides the victory.

—*General George C. Marshall*

He . . . got the
better of himself,
and that's the best
kind of victory one
can wish for.

—*Miguel de Cervantes*

MIND AND MUSCLE

"Football is played, above all, with the heart and mind," said Pennsylvania State University Coach Joe Paterno. "It's played with the body only secondarily. A coach's first duty is to coach minds. If he doesn't succeed at that, his team will not reach its potential."[1]

If football and other sports are played with the mind, is it possible to program the mind for victory? Can hypnosis, with proper suggestions, turn a loser into a winner by the power of the mind?

Les Cunningham, Ph. D., Australian hypnotherapist, has used hypnosis to improve the performance of many athletes. He suspects that the use of hypnosis lies behind much of the success of Soviet-bloc athletes in Olympic competition.

I was a pool player for many years, and I have used hypnosis to improve my performance at the pool table. Later in this chapter, I will describe how I've worked with some pool players to remove the deep-seated subconscious factors that were hindering their games.

But let's get something straight at the outset: Hypnosis will not turn a Joe Garagiola into a Joe DiMaggio. It will not turn a weekend pool-hall patron into a Wimpy Lassiter or a Mike Sigel. Enabling the couch potato to rise from the sofa and run the marathon takes an act of God not hypnotic suggestion.

Hypnosis should not be used to help someone ignore an injury and perform to maximum capacity. Ignoring an injury for the sake of temporary gain can make the injury permanent, or worse. But hypnosis can help you to get the most out of yourself which, as Cervantes wrote, is the best kind of victory one can hope for.

Even those who might never have thought of hypnosis have acknowledged that muscle alone doesn't win the athletic event. Sports history is populated with names of players whose physical abilities were mediocre but whose mental attitudes spurred them and their teams to victory. Billy Ripken of the Baltimore Orioles might not possess the physical talent of Cal, his brother and teammate. But his hustle and determination have earned him a respected niche among major-league infielders. Billy Martin, whose fiery personality led the New York Yankees and Oakland Athletics to championships under his managership, was a spark plug as a player, too. But it was his competitive attitude, not his physical prowess, that made the difference on the field. Leo Durocher, who achieved greatness as a manager, also enjoyed a playing career marked by heads-up play that compensated for lack of physical talent.

Durocher took the field with a single-minded determination to win. He once remarked:

> What are we out at the park for except to win? I'd trip my mother. I'll help her up, brush her off, tell her I'm sorry. But mother don't make it to third.[2]

"We become what we think we are," wrote Les Cunningham in his book, *Hypnosport: How You Can Improve Your Sporting Performances.* "If we think of success, we become successful. If we think of failure, we become failures."[3]

They *Expected* to Score

That was the attitude Paterno tried to communicate to his players. He took a dim view of end-zone theatrics after a touchdown. "When a Nittany Lion scores a touchdown," he said, "he doesn't dance and go berserk in the end zone. When a Penn Stater goes on that field, he expects to make a touchdown."[4]

Paterno knew that a winning coach must also cultivate a winning attitude, and he saw Bear Bryant of the University of Alabama as the epitome of confidence:

> When Bear Bryant . . . walked out on that football field, self-confidence hung in the air around him like a fine mist. That was worth at least one touchdown for Alabama.[5]

And Paterno saw himself as a winner. He wasn't content to see himself as a good coach, or the Coach of the Year, or even the best coach in Penn State history. "I didn't see why I should leave room in the number one spot for sharing with Bear Bryant or Vince Lombardi or anybody else,"[6] he declared.

The mother of Olympic runner Brenda Morehead urged the same type of attitude when she advised her daughter, "Don't want to win; want a record!"[7] Whether Morehead set the record or fell short of it, that confident determination propelled her to victory in the Olympics.

If you believe you will succeed, you will succeed. If you believe you will fail, you will fail. Imagination is a powerful tool for accomplishment. If you can produce vivid images of success in your mind, those images penetrate to your subconscious, and from there they can light your way to success.

I know this is easy to say. I do not want to oversimplify or mislead you into thinking that programming your subconscious mind for success in a competitive sport is as easy as sinking a four-inch putt or getting on first by taking four straight balls. Besides determination and ability, many factors contribute. Hypnosis, self-suggestion, and hypnoanalysis can, however, make a tremendous difference with a motivated person, as you shall see.

Willie's Prayer: 'Don't Let It Be Me'

In the final game of the 1951 National League playoffs, the New York Giants were fortunate that Bobby Thomson came through at the crucial moment. With one out in the ninth inning, Thomson represented the winning run for the Giants. Thomson confidently strode to the plate and knocked a Ralph Branca pitch out of the park, making the Giants the National League champions.

The man scheduled to hit behind Thomson was a rookie named Willie Mays. Mays was in the on-deck circle praying. His prayer was not, "Please God, let Bobby get a hit so we can go to the World Series." It was, "Please don't let it be me. Don't let me come to bat now, God."[8]

Would Willie have come through in the clutch? Not likely. He was 1 for 10 in the playoffs, and at the time was totally lacking in confidence.

Later, it was a different story. Manager Leo Durocher took Willie under his wing and, over time, instilled confidence in the youngster. At one point, when Willie was moping around in the clubhouse, feeling sorry for himself because of his poor batting performance, Durocher told him:

> You're the greatest ball player I ever saw or ever hope to see. . . . You can hit it into the bleachers here, over the fence, anywhere you want. . . .[9]

Willie, of course, went on to live up to Durocher's prescient description. Had he possessed the confidence in 1951 that he acquired in later years, he would have been praying for a chance to come to bat.

Durocher's challenge was to get the negative, pessimistic thinking out of Mays' subconscious mind and replace it with positive, optimistic thinking. The manager succeeded through patient reassurance and reinforcement. A hypnoanalyst might have done it more quickly. Had Willie used hypnosis to purge the image of failure from his subconscious, the Giants might not have needed a dramatic stretch drive and a cliff-hanger playoff series to win the pennant.

"Boundless confidence seems to ride hand-in-hand with the success of an individual or a team," says Cunningham in the preface to his book.

Was it pure luck that Babe Ruth, after calling two strikes on himself, was able to point toward the stands, then drive a home run within a few feet of where he had pointed? Not likely. The Babe had superb confidence in himself and that confidence gave him the poise, timing, and concentration to accomplish what he aimed to accomplish.

THE PYRAMID OF SUCCESS

Cunningham compares sporting success to a pyramid. Its triangular base consists of three factors: intelligence, physical conditioning, and psychological conditioning.[10] The athlete achieves peak performance when all three factors are in fine harmony.

A good coach can provide the extra intelligence. The coach's knowledge, training, and experience serve as guides to setting up schedules for training and competition. The tennis player who schedules too many tournaments and not enough training sessions is unlikely to make it to Wimbledon. The one whose schedule brings the athlete to the tournament in peak form is the one most likely to win.

Once those schedules are set, the athlete has to stick with them. This calls for discipline. The athlete has to see the schedule of training and com petition as a road to success. With that road clearly fixed in mind, the competitor embarks on it with single-minded determination.

Physical conditioning is the next prerequisite to athletic success. As Cunningham notes, a good strong competitor will always beat an equally good but slightly weaker opponent.[11] When athletes in training see themselves getting stronger and fitter, they receive good, positive reinforcement.

Finally comes the psychological conditioning—the mental programming for success. Self-hypnosis can be an effective tool for this programming. Through it, athletes can learn, in Cunningham's words, "to imagine with crystal clarity" the points on the pathways they have mapped out."[12]

Cunningham divides his inputs into three overlapping stages: long term, medium term and short term. Long-term strategy begins before the season starts. With the help of self-hypnosis, the athlete can concentrate on the ultimate goal. Cunningham observes:

> At no time should negative thoughts or doubts be allowed to intrude into your imaginings. The only things to think about are positive steps toward the championship. Visions of the crowd, the arena, the sights, sounds and smells, your role in the winning play, the championship-winning perfor-

> mance, the applause and the euphoria associated with victories should be all that concerns you at this stage in your preparation.[13]

During the training period, Cunningham urges athletes to go into self-hypnosis and imagine themselves growing in strength, coordination and stamina.[14]

As the day of competition approaches, medium-term and short-term preparations begin. Then, athletes practice and perfect the correct style. At this stage they can, under self-hypnosis, see themselves performing the correct way. They can feel the correct grip on the bat, the club, or the racquet. They can imagine themselves swimming with the correct stroke.

On the eve of the contest, athletes may experience stage fright. If they know how to use self-hypnosis, they can overcome this by imagining in vivid detail all the events of the day before the contest. They should start doing this a week in advance. If possible, they should plan a routine to be followed that day and stick to it. They should imagine what they will be eating, feel themselves experiencing the pleasant tiredness, then sinking into a comfortable night's sleep. If insomnia sets in, they can use self-hypnosis to relax themselves and fall asleep.

Several hours before the contest, or even just before the contest, they can relax themselves through self-hypnosis. After taking last-minute instructions from the coach, they can visualize how the contest will go. They can see themselves performing at top level, their muscles perfectly tuned, their reflexes sharp, their energy fully mobilized.

Peak performance demands an appropriate level of arousal. The rule of thumb is that the simpler the task, the higher the level of arousal necessary to accomplish it. Cunningham suggests that players associate different levels of arousal with different colors.[15] By concentrating on the appropriate color, they can thus achieve the proper level of arousal at the proper time. Self-hypnosis is one way of achieving the desired state of arousal at will.

When the mind is properly *programmed*, the athlete goes into the contest confident, poised, and devoid of negative thoughts. This confidence does not remove the possibility of mistakes or bad bounces or bad calls by the referee. But it insulates the player from the demoralizing effects of these breaks. The tennis player who makes a bad serve during a match will not be rattled by the mistake. The player with positive programming knows that one bad serve doesn't lose a tournament.

Nor should we expect that the athlete who uses hypnosis will never lose. Remember that no baseball team has ever won a pennant with a perfect season. You win some, lose some, and some get rained out. But athletes who are programmed for victory will not be deterred by the defeats along the way. They will learn from their defeats and, thus, turn them into positive experiences.

To be a success, you have to concentrate your entire mind on being a success. When excellent pianists play, they concentrate their entire minds on playing the piano. They're not wondering whether, maybe, they'll hit the wrong note. An excellent pilot, when flying a plane, concentrates entirely on piloting the aircraft. It won't do to concentrate partly on piloting the plane and partly on the fear of not doing it right. Self-consciousness is anathema to the pianist, the pilot, and the athlete.

When a 14-year-old girl from San Francisco swam the English Channel, she concentrated her mind entirely on the challenge she faced. Her concentration was so intense that, mentally, she had already swum the channel in advance, before she ever got into the water. It was an accomplished fact before she ever began. She became the youngest person ever to swim the English channel, and she did it under self-hypnosis. Had part of her mind been concentrated on the fear of what might happen if she didn't make it, then she would have been sapping her own strength, causing self-defeating feelings and thoughts.

HOW WE SAP OUR STRENGTH

The truth of the matter is that we all sap our own strength to a certain extent, depending on the amount of fear we allow to creep into our minds. We even get afraid to let go of our fear. We think maybe fear is a good thing; maybe it motivates us. We may think, "Maybe if I'm afraid I'm going to be poor, then I'll have to strive to be rich; maybe if I'm afraid I'm going to lose the game, I'll play better." But nothing could be farther from the truth. When can you accomplish what you want to do? The answer is when you get rid of the fear that you might not accomplish it. Remember: Fear creates that which one is afraid of.

Three negative emotions must be eliminated before you can get started toward becoming a better athlete. Hynoanalysts call them the "unholy triumvirate": fear, anxiety, and guilt. They do no good; they hold you back. Before you can remove them, you have to learn to recognize them, so that you can keep them from moving back in.

The first and biggest negative emotion is fear. It usually creeps back in the form of motivation. You say, "Oh, it's good for me to be afraid; it motivates me." But that's ridiculous. Fear motivates people to panic. The only limitation to free speech that Justice Hugo Black would admit is that classic premise of Justice Oliver Wendell Holmes: Nobody has a right to yell fire in a crowded theater when there is no fire. Why? Because it makes people afraid. They panic. They lose their reason. They rush for the exit, even though it's blocked. Emotion comes to the door and reason flies out the window. Whatever you're afraid of, it must go.

The next negative emotion is anxiety, or worry. Business people worry, and that gives them ulcers. All successful people have ulcers, right? Far from it. The really successful people handle their business without ulcers. The amount of energy you're using to make the ulcers, to get the stomach to secrete the acid, is working against you, not for you. That means you're sublimating other drives, such as hostility, by injuring yourself. Fear and anxiety are negative emotions that injure you. Channel the hostility into the business itself.

The most insidious of all the negative emotions is guilt. Guilt is an after-the-fact emotion. You feel guilty because you made the wrong decision; therefore, you punish yourself. You feel guilty because of your childhood or because of something that happened a long time ago. You didn't do the best for your mother or your father, or for your brother or your sister; or you could have done this, or you could have done that. The guilt makes you certain that you don't deserve to be a success. Therefore, if you don't deserve to be a success, you must find a way to avoid success. This all happens on a subconscious level.

Guilt tells you that you don't deserve to win. It calls for punishment. How can you punish yourself? By never achieving the goals for which you are striving, by never winning. Clearly, you can do without fear, anxiety, and guilt.

Guilt In Action

A 37-year-old pool player was having difficulty sinking the winning ball when in competition. His only symptom was his shaking arm. Once his concentration became broken by the shaking, he would then worry and frequently miss the winning ball.

In hypnoanalysis, he recalled a time at the age of 15 when he was losing a pool game and tried to win it by cheating. His opponent caught him. To save face, he beat up his opponent and was barred from the facility for six months. The guilt brought on by the cheating and by the beating of his opponent led him to punish himself. He hated himself for the way he acted and decided he shouldn't win any more.

Once we brought this scene into his consciousness, the player realized that it wasn't within his jurisdiction to punish himself. He let go of his self-hate and his tendency toward self-punishment.

After I have cleared the negative emotions from the subconscious, I replace them with 14 principles, developed by hypnoanalysts in the past,[16] that all successful winners in every category in every walk of life must have:

1. Everything will work out okay.

2. You will have enough time to fulfill your goal.

3. You will be able to acquire the necessary power to do what you need to do.

4. You can acquire the necessary knowledge to complete your goal.

5. Over the long haul, good thoughts prevail.

6. You believe in being merciful, and that means winning quickly.

7. You believe the whole world in which you compete is within your personal domination.

8. You believe that you deserve to win wherever you play.

9. You believe in yourself and in your ability to overcome your obstacles.

10. Winners love themselves. You love yourself.

11. Winners always feel as if they've won, even if they've lost, because they've learned something.

12. Winners avoid self-indulgent, victimlike feelings. The world loves a winner.

13. When you are playing, you are no longer aware of yourself. You seem to lose yourself completely in your play.

14. Relax and win.

Both Tim Gallwey, author of *The Inner Game of Tennis*[17] and coauthors James M. Rippe, M.D., and William Southmayd, M.D., of *The Sports Performance Factors*[18] emphasize that the body/mind has a wisdom of its own, that it can execute extremely coordinated movements of all kinds on its own without thinking or being told how to do them. This so-called wisdom of the body is actually the subconscious in action, which remains unrelied on due to thoughts of the "should" or "ought-to" nature overriding the subconscious, mind/body know-how. Consequently, in hypnoanalysis, I remove the negativity first, the district of one's own mind/body second, and then implant the subconscious positive suggestions.

Beating the Voodoo Hex

A fellow hypnoanalyst, Dr. Earl Taylor, used hypnotherapy to bring a major-league baseball player out of a batting slump.[19] The player—we'll call him Slugger—had grown up in a big-city ghetto in a strongly religious environment. When three new players from the Caribbean joined the club, they told him they had put a voodoo hex on him. His batting average then began to plummet.

Dr. Taylor found a number of negative experiences in Slugger's background. Here are two of them:

1. When he was in high school, he discovered that the woman he thought was his mother was actually his grandmother. He had been led to believe that his real mother was his sister. When he discovered the truth, he had felt abandoned. This was the symptom-producing event.

2. The initial sensitizing event came earlier. When he was a boy, he got into a fight with another child. Slugger was a big kid, and he hit his opponent so hard he thought he had killed him.

Now Slugger was in the big leagues. He had a million-dollar contract, was married and had a couple of children. But his bat and glove were not the only things he was carrying onto the field. He was also carrying a bag of guilt. He hadn't been paying enough attention to his family. He had the residual guilt over the time he thought he had killed a boy. This made him susceptible to the suggestion that he was about to become the victim of a voodoo hex.

Dr. Taylor identified the problem. Through regression under hypnosis, he helped Slugger analyze the cause of his problem. The fears were located and removed.

The day after his first treatment, Slugger went three for four at the plate. He was later traded to another team, but he stayed in touch with Dr. Taylor. On one occasion, Dr. Taylor hypnotized him over the telephone, telling him he would have a wonderful day at bat. Slugger came to bat with the bases loaded and drove the ball into the stands.

NEGATIVE THOUGHTS IN THE CORNER POCKET

My interest in pool has led me to develop a program for helping pool players through hypnosis. I offer a week-long, intensive-subconscious analysis to pool players. This helps me to analyze their subconscious minds and find out exactly what is happening to cause problems with their pool playing. Sometimes, the thing interfering with the pool game is something that is interfering with the person's happiness in other areas of life.

Hank Wanted to Play

One player who came to me was Hank, a 43-year-old self-employed contractor from Minnesota. "The problem is that I don't make all the balls I am supposed to make," Hank said. "It is extremely difficult for me to run a rack [sink 9 to 15 balls consecutively]. Sometimes I can run four or five balls. It's very frustrating."

Hank had operated a pool hall for about five years after graduating from high school. That had been about 15 years ago.

"One of the reasons I quit was that I wasn't getting any better," he said.

I asked him how long his playing had been a problem.

"Probably ever since the first few years," he said. As we talked, he told me: "I think I know why. I think I have a problem with embarrassment."

Hank told me the embarrassment is compounded by the fact that he likes to play with his friends watching. "I don't enjoy it unless people are watching; nobody watching is what makes it worse," he said. Yet, he told me, he gets embarrassed and feels stupid when he misses a shot. In other words, Hank plays for people's approval.

"What makes it better," I asked.

"When I am really in my element. People watching, and playing for a lot of money."

"What could you do, if you were cured, that you can't do now?" I asked.

"I am probably, even now, capable of being the best player in my town if I can only make the balls I am supposed to make. I want to run a rack and I want to run out and I can't."

If you're not a pool enthusiast, you may need a little explanation here. There are certain shots that a pool player at a given level should be able to make without too much difficulty. They're shots the player has made hundreds of times before. Hank was missing the shots he should have been making.

Hank plays a game called Nine Ball—the game Tom Cruise played in the movie *The Color of Money*. The object in Nine Ball is to sink the balls in succession, starting with the one ball and going through the nine ball. The player who sinks the nine ball is the winner. When Hank refers to "running out," he means dropping the balls in succession, including the nine ball for the victory.

The number five seemed to be significant for Hank. He told me he had been divorced five years. When I asked him about his friends, he said he had had four or five over the past few years. He said he had enjoyed good sex except for about four or five times. He had five children.

Hank had enjoyed an "extremely happy" childhood.

No Responsibilities

"I played all the time and had no responsibilities," he said. "It ruined me as an adult. I could do anything I wanted." How many of us can do anything we want?

I asked about his father. Hank didn't like him very much. "The last time I saw him, I was five or six." His parents had divorced when he was an infant.

We were looking at some stuck places. The word-association test was revealing. Here's how it went:

Ryan: When I grow up . . .
Hank: I'll be a star.
Ryan: I would rather ________ than win.
Hank: Play.
Ryan: In order to survive . . .
Hank: I must play.
Ryan: I don't want to grow up because . . .
Hank: Of responsibilities.
Ryan: Punishment . . .
Hank: Discipline.
Ryan: I punish myself because . . .
Hank: I don't like it.
Ryan: Seeing things through . . .
Hank: Accomplishment.

The word-association test made this clear: Winning at pool wasn't the important thing to Hank. The important thing was playing. Playing all the time is something little kids do. So like a child, Hank had been playing for people's approval. He wasn't really taking the game seriously, though that's what he wanted to do.

When I told Hank he had a Ponce de Leon syndrome, he accepted it. Being a carefree child had been delightful. Accepting the responsibilities of adulthood had been painful.

Hank had married the high-school homecoming queen, but life didn't have a storybook ending. He was still a child, emotionally, in no position to handle a marriage. He was never home; he was always playing pool. Then came the divorce.

"For the next three or four years, all I wanted was the money in the pocket. Now that I am going back to pool, the subconscious is saying, 'This is death.' Pool is worse than cancer."

In his mind, Hank associated pool playing with a negative period in his life. He believed that to be good at pool was worse than death, and his identity was tied up in what he did.

I regressed him several times and followed his feelings when he was playing pool back to his childhood. I helped him to relieve those feelings in those stuck places, then move on.

In about his 10th session, he said, "I think yesterday was terrific; I still feel like a kid. The problem is this death thing, not the child thing. During the time when I was playing, it was horrible. For about three years, no one knew where I was. If my subconscious believes pool is bad, then I'm not going to do it."

I helped him relieve those negative suggestions and to break this bond of identity between pool and his bad feelings. We reviewed some of his negative attitudes about God, religion, and punishment. I helped him identify the areas he needed to grow up in, and other areas in which he needed to take care of himself. I gave him many positive suggestions and made a tape of those suggestions for him to take home.

In his last session, Hank told me he was feeling "super." He felt very satisfied with his analysis.

Inhibited by Low Self-esteem

Alicia wanted to become a world-champion pool player, and she came all the way from Alaska to get help from me. Pool filled a space in her life that had been empty since her divorce.

"I'm addicted to it," the 40-year-old woman told me. But her game was suffering because she couldn't concentrate on her playing.

"Sometimes your mind is thinking about so many different things that you are trying too hard," she said. She would become tense, her arm would tighten up, and she would miss the shots she should have been able to make with ease.

"I want to sort things out and get the direction that I need to get rid of my inhibitions," she said. "I'm always concerned about what people are thinking and my low self-esteem."

I learned that Alicia was an adult child of an alcoholic and had been through a number of terrible experiences. She was raped twice. Her father had abused her. A boyfriend had left her while she was pregnant.

The word-association test showed that Alicia felt stuck at the age of 16—about the age at which she was first raped. She said she lived "in a fairy-tale world" and did not want to grow up. We were again dealing with the Ponce de Leon syndrome.

I regressed her to the womb and found the initial sensitizing event. It was birth itself. She had felt comfortable and secure in the womb. But as the time for birth approached, things got scary. She wasn't eager to be separated from her mother. In the here and now, that translated into a scare each time she got close to someone, or any time there were changes in her life. It also got scary when she began to play pool really well.

So Alicia was afraid of change. Growing up meant changing and that was scary for her. She had already experienced several unpleasant changes. Once we removed this negativity from her subconscious and raised her self-esteem, she was ready to return to Alaska and polish her pool game. I gave her the name of a doctor in Fairbanks and urged her to continue her treatment.

Alicia was suffering from two of the biggest problems in sports: fear and lack of concentration. Once we identify the initial sensitizing event, the problem usually resolves itself. The fear is removed.

Lack of concentration is another matter. I have worked with several golfers who have this problem. For many people, it's simply a matter of learning how to concentrate and how to focus all their energy on what they're doing.

But for other people, concentration can be disrupted by feelings of guilt, anxiety, anger, and other negative emotions. Frequently, self-hypnosis will free a person from these feelings and open the door to concentration.

Blowing It under Pressure

Cliff, a 28-year-old Californian, was another pool player with a problem. "I play a decent game of pool until I get under pressure," he said. "I talk myself out of it, it seems. More often than not, I lose it. I just start losing my confidence. I doubt myself; I feel a lot of embarrassment if I miss it."

How long had this been a problem?

"Forever, I guess. When I was younger—at 15 or 16—I don't think it bothered me. I've only started going to tournaments for the last two years."

What makes it worse?

"When I want to win."

What makes it better?

"I don't know. I still play a good game around the guys I have known all my life. But the closer I get to the money spot, the more I start dogging it. Then I feel the pressure."

I asked what he would be able to do once the problem was solved that he couldn't do now. His reply, "It stops me from winning. I blow it."

This was an easy case to work on. Cliff said he played a decent game until he was under pressure. In his first sentence, his subconscious mind tipped me off to what I was looking for. I wanted to find his very first experience with pressure and how it was associated with pool.

"More often that not," he said, "I lose it." I knew enough about this sort of thing to guess that he had experienced a birth trauma.

Here's how his word-association test went:

RYAN: Life . . .
CLIFF: Live.
RYAN: Death . . .
CLIFF: Live.

So life is like death. I say live and he says die. So he has had some death suggestion. The test continued:

RYAN: The real problem is . . .
CLIFF: Nervous.
RYAN: Insecurity . . .
CLIFF: Nervousness.
RYAN: Pressure feels like . . .
CLIFF: Nervousness.

So insecurity, nervousness, and pressure are synonymous with each other, and with his problem. The real problem equals nervousness, anxiety, and insecurity. The test continued:

Ryan: Embarrassment feels like . . .
Cliff: Shame.
Ryan: Underneath it all . . .
Cliff: I am ashamed.

When Cliff would get close to winning, he would begin to doubt himself, feel ashamed, feel the pressure, and blow the shot.

Ryan: Doubt begins . . .
Cliff: When I'm close to winning.
Ryan: Complete a sentence that starts with the word "who."
Cliff: Who am I?

Cliff has an identity problem.

Ryan: Sometimes I feel I am stuck at age . . .
Cliff: Twelve.
Ryan: I punish . . .
Cliff: Myself.
Ryan: I have always been ashamed . . .
Cliff: For wishing bad things on my friends.
Ryan: My punishment is . . .
Cliff: Losing concentration.
Ryan: It all started . . .
Cliff: When I was a kid.
Ryan: It got worse when . . .
Cliff: I got well.

So here's where we were: Cliff felt very much that he didn't know who he was. At the very bottom of it all, he was scared. He was punishing himself for something he had done a long time ago. He was also punishing himself for wishing bad things on some of his friends. His punishment was his loss of concentration.

When I explained this to him, he got excited and agreed that it sounded reasonable. I did a dream analysis. Here's what Cliff dreamed:

> A white wall was standing by itself with black words written on it. As I walked toward it, trying to read it, I was almost ready to make out the words when the wall fell backwards.

Here's how we interpreted the dream: The wall, with the writing on it, was keeping him from doing well. He was going to get well and solve the problem. The feeling he associated with the dream was connected to a scene when he was about 12 years old and was in a car with friends. He had two groups of friends. He didn't know how to choose between the two groups. He wasn't sure how people felt about him. He had a lot of mixed emotions. He kept telling himself to "quit giving a shit."

To help him improve his pool game, we had to make him see that he wasn't playing pool to please anybody. The 12-year-old did not have to choose among friends. When he was playing pool, he was playing an opponent. If that opponent was a friend, he did not have to choose between winning the game and keeping his friend. He could do both.

Subsequently, I searched through his subconscious looking for "the pressure." Lo and behold, we were back at birth.

As he remembered emerging from the womb, he said, "I don't want to go through it. I'm scared, I guess . . . I can feel the pressure. It's closing in all around me."

Under hypnosis, Cliff realized that he felt this same kind of feeling during his pool game. Things were closing in around him and he didn't want to do it. The pressure in a pool game tipped off his subconscious mind: He didn't want to be born; pressure from playing pool was like being born; consequently, he didn't want to play pool. We wiped that out, completely removing it from his subconscious and desensitizing his mind to the feeling of being pushed out of the womb when he wasn't really ready.

In a subsequent session, we learned more about the guilt feelings from wishing bad things on his friends. Cliff had a friend who had mistakenly hurt him. Cliff had wished a lot of bad things on his friend. The friend died when he was about 16.

The guilt from this experience spilled into his pool game. When he was playing pool, he was wishing for the other person to lose. It would trigger his guilt feelings over his dead friend. We talked about that, and he was able to separate his pool game from the guilt feelings.

In his 14th and final session, he said, "I am ready to go out and compete." He did.

LOSING CAN BE POSITIVE

To go out and compete isn't the same thing as to go out and win. I can't hypnotize you into winning every time, and you certainly can't hypnotize yourself into becoming an invariable winner. But you can learn to convert losing into a positive experience.

Will Rogers has been quoted as saying, "Everything is funny as long as it is happening to somebody else." Losing is a lot easier to take if it's the other person who is doing the losing. For most Americans, the word "lose" is a cussword, a four-letter obscenity that ranks up there with obscene descriptions of bodily functions and parts.

We're a success-obsessed culture. Only dieters and masochists enjoy losing. Yet, for every player who wins a tournament, there's at least one who loses. While most of us would rather go to hell than admit it, we lose more than we win.

Winning and losing are both part of the human predicament, but the first is vastly more popular than the last. Losing is so undervalued that most people would rather pretend it doesn't exist. They would like to wish it into oblivion.

Somewhere back there, the win-at-all-costs attitude became the American religion. Vince Lombardi gave this religion it's Golden Rule: "Winning isn't everything; it's the only thing." By making winning the only thing, we make dropouts of people who are capable of contributing to our society.

Since there are only so many places at the top and there's such fierce competition to get to them, many will lose. Then what?

FAILURE: A "CRIME" THAT PAYS

"Failure seems to be regarded as the one unpardonable crime, success as the all-redeeming virtue," lamented nineteenth-century statesman Charles Adams. Conventional wisdom tells us crime doesn't pay. But if losing is a crime, there is a payoff in increased self-knowledge. In the 1979 Sugar Bowl, with the national championship at stake against Alabama, Joe Paterno called for a run on a goal-line play when his gut instinct told him to go for the pass. Penn State lost. Four years later, again in the Sugar Bowl and again with the national championship at stake, Paterno's gut told him to pass on a key play for short yardage against Georgia. Remembering 1979, he called for the pass. The play worked, and Paterno had a national championship, thanks to a bit of self-knowledge gained in defeat.

As I write this, two people come to mind who, by most appearances, were very fortunate men, and winners to boot: W.C. Fields and Mark Twain.

I remember W. C. Fields from two hilarious movie scenes involving the game of pool. In one, he rolled the cue ball around by running the cue along the top of the ball. In another he used a crooked cue.

Fields was a masterful comedic actor. Was he successful? You could say so. He certainly won fortune and acclaim. But the consensus was that he was an alcoholic.

Did he enjoy pleasing people with his comedy? He once said, "I am free of prejudices. I hate everyone equally." The "everyone" must have included himself.

Mark Twain? Fantastically talented author and humorist, who also was a billiards buff. Was he a success? Twain wrote, "Byron despised the human race because he despised himself. I feel as Byron did, and for the same reason." He also wrote, "We all feel inferior, just about different things."

Twain was famous, but was he a winner?

History, literature, and folklore spill out famous losers: Romeo and Juliet, Shakespeare's losers in the game of love; the fabulous Casey, who left Mudville without joy when he struck out with the bases loaded in the ninth; General George Custer, a dandy of a general until he met his Waterloo at the Battle of the Little Big Horn; Adolf Hitler, whose book *Mein Kampf* drew a blueprint for a reich that was to last for 1,000 years but died in its 12th year amid the rubble of a collapsing empire. And how about Robin Hood the bandit, Davy Crockett and his fellow losers at the Alamo; and Christopher Columbus, who failed to find a new trade route to India but unknowingly stumbled across a new world? From an earthly standpoint, even Jesus Christ was a loser: He had no permanent home, no permanent job, and no extensive religious organization. He died ignominiously as a criminal, accused of sedition against the Roman empire and blasphemy against the very God in whose name he spoke.

Not everyone can be a famous loser, and how many of the just-named people would you trade places with if you could? I wouldn't trade my life with a single one. So why even examine the subject of losing? Several things about losing are worth considering.

First of all, losing a game isn't such a fearful thing once you've faced the fear squarely. Today's loser can be tomorrow's champion. "There's always next year" is one of the most hallowed and comforting expressions in the world of sports.

Far more important than the objective fact of winning and losing is your subjective judgment of your own performance. Regardless of how others rate your performance, if you do not measure up to your own standards, then you tend to think of yourself as a failure.

As Les Cunningham expressed it, "Remember, the whole world can classify you as a failure, but you never become one until you admit it to yourself."[20]

People often use a double standard in rating their performances against the performances of others. They will be tolerant of the errors and shortcomings of others, yet hold themselves to the most exacting standards. Remember this standard from the chapter on public speaking.

Many explanations have been advanced for this phenomenon. The point I want to make is simply this: Take a look at your performance and learn as much as you can from your losing as well as from your winning.

Eric Berne, the author of *What Do You Say after You Say Hello?* and *Games People Play,* said, "A winner knows what he'll do if he loses, but doesn't talk about it; whereas a loser doesn't know what he'll do if he loses, and only talks about what he'll do if he wins."[21]

Along Berne's lines, here are a few ways to think about losing, as paraphrased from Les Cunningham:

- Life is a gamble. If you don't risk losing, you have no chance of winning. If you can eliminate the fear of losing, you can increase substantially your chance of winning because the mind is focused on the task, not on the feeling.
- If you never lose, you can't appreciate winning. Without losing, the competition would be meaningless. If you won all the time, competing would soon become boring, and you'd take up something more challenging in which you run the risk of losing. You need to lose occasionally just to feel the exhilaration of winning.
- Competition can be enjoyable in itself. It can motivate you to play a better game and surpass yourself, to transcend your limitations in some way. This can yield much satisfaction and fun.
- Learning to lose will help you overcome failure. If you understand the cause of your loss, you will be motivated to avoid that cause in the future.
- You can improve your performance by playing opponents who play better than you do. Losing to a better player can push you to greater achievements. It's more gratifying to lose to a better player than to beat a player of inferior ability.

Key Concepts

- Sports are played with the mind as well as the muscles. Athletic success is built upon a pyramid, the base of which consists of physical conditioning, psychological conditioning, and intelligence.
- Psychological conditioning is done in three stages: long term, medium term, and short term. Long-term conditioning starts in the preseason or at the beginning of training with positive suggestions to the subconscious and total avoidance of negative thinking. Thoughts of fear, anxiety, and guilt must be banished. In the medium term, athletes should imagine themselves growing stronger as training progresses, executing plays and developing their techniques perfectly. In the short term, they should use positive suggestions to overcome stage fright and to bring themselves to the proper state of arousal. Self-hypnosis is helpful at each of these stages.
- The mind, programmed for victory, will not be defeated by temporary setbacks such as a poor serve, an error in the field, or a fumble. It will learn from the mistake and renew its determination to win.
- Self-hypnosis should not be used to suggest that the athlete ignore injuries.
- Athletes should realize that no one wins all the time. The important thing is to perform to your maximum potential and to learn from your losses.

Growth Exercise

1. List the options for your pyramid of success.
   a. Physical conditioning ______________________________
   b. Psychological conditioning ______________________________
   c. Intelligence ______________________________

2. Are you satisfied with what you have? If not, what are you willing to do?

   ____

   ____

3. Plan your long-, medium- and short-term psychological conditioning.

   ____

   ____

   ____

4. Make a list of what you learn from every loss.

   ____

   ____

5. List the criteria you use to judge your own sports performance? How does it compare to the criteria by which you judge others?

   ____

   ____

   ____

6. Psychologist Fritz Perls once said, "The human species has the unique distinction of being the only species on the planet that is capable of interfering with its own growth." Review the ideas in this chapter and list the ways in which you get in the way of your own sports performance.

   ____

   ____

   ____

CHAPTER TWELVE

GOD IS NOT IN CONTROL!

God is creative energy.
That we experience this energy
as love,
that within us it promotes order,
happiness, life-energy,
and all other things
that we feel as "good,"
that we can receive this energy
from those close to us
and pass it on to others,
is simple enough
and easy to discuss consciously
with depressed people
or those with behavior problems
resulting from depression.

—Thomas A Ritzman, M.D.

AT SOME TIME, WE ALL ASK: WHO OR WHAT IS GOD?

Self-image shapes reality! Intimately connected to self-image and self-esteem, frequently unconsciously, lies our conception of God. Very often in my practice, patients report symptoms of depression, low self-esteem, chronic guilt, and codependency. I find that in about half the cases the subconscious root of the problem involves God—who or what He or She is. This involves the concept of God as judge, jury, and executioner, or as a loving father figure.

People are plagued by such questions as "Who is God?" "What's He like?" "What does He expect of me?" "What is sin, really?" "Am I guilty of sin against God?" "What is my punishment?"

In Old Testament times, we heard directly from God, according to our Judeo-Christian heritage. He talked to us through a sort of hallucinated voice. The Ten Commandments were received directly from God.

Between 1000 and 300 B.C., the concept of consciousness developed, and we stopped listening to the part of our minds that would hallucinate voices. We now think of God as being in heaven or within us and guiding us from inside through prayer—not as a hallucinated voice.

As Dr. Gerald May said in *Care of Mind—Care of Spirit*:

> From the time of Christ until well after the Reformation, little differentiation was made between psychological and spiritual disorders. . . . With the advent of Freudian psychoanalysis, however, drastic changes began to take place. . . . Today's secular psychology addresses a great deal about how we come to be the way we are. . . . However, it can offer nothing in terms of why we exist or how we should use our lives.[1]

One reason for this lack may be the difference in spiritual alignment between therapists and their clients. Dr. Daniel Zelling reported in the *American Journal of Psychiatry* that 95 percent of Americans polled believe in God, compared with 5 percent of the members of the American Psychiatric Association and 43 percent of the American Psychological Association.[2] So well over half of the care providers are, in effect, denying God or the role of spirituality to those who seek treatment. This could account for the lack of success secular psychotherapists have had in treating spiritual problems.

C. Alan Anderson, Ph.D., cites an experiment at the University of Redlands in California in which the effectiveness of prayer therapy was compared with that of psychotherapy. The subjects in prayer therapy showed a 72 percent degree of improvement while those in psychotherapy showed only 67 percent improvement. Those praying in only a random way experienced no improvement.

One reason prayers may seem to go unanswered is that they are not directed toward the individual's real needs. Until we confront our true needs, we cannot pray effectively. The participants in prayer therapy were subjected first to psychological testing to determine their weaknesses—the matters needing attention in prayer. Most participants were plagued by those familiar villains: fear, guilt, inferiority feelings, and misguided love (which is hate in disguise).[3] These are precisely the villains that hypnoanalysis is so helpful in unmasking. And if hypnoanalysis is to help patients come to terms with who and what God is, it goes without saying that the hypnoanalyst must believe in and have a reverence toward God.

From the outset, let me emphasize that there is only one God, regardless of what religion one believes in.

In his book *The Problem Is God*, C. Alan Anderson quotes an unnamed scholar, "Rightly understood, the problem of God is not one problem among several others; it is the only problem there is."

Anderson comments, "The problem of God is so all-embracing that everything else must be seen in relation to it."

I support this idea, yet in about 50 percent of the cases I see, the GOD problem looms very large.

I believe there are two broad categories in which God is viewed. These categories are not along any religious lines because my experience indicates that people from the same religious background will view God from different angles.

My work has shown that God is subconsciously thought of as either love or as a parent figure. These two simple classifications illustrate my point, although I realize many volumes have been written about God. For my purpose, living in a largely Judeo-Christian culture, this simplification works.

If God is love, then the believer feels loved by God, has freedom, takes responsibility for self, and doesn't blame God for circumstances in the world. If God is a parent figure, then God is judge, jury, and executioner. The personal believer feels wrong, guilty, enslaved, and insecure. God then is anthropomorphic. God is created in the image and likeness of man and not the reverse. I believe that God is love, and since love is a feeling, then God is a feeling.

From this standpoint, I attempt to help people feel that feeling of God, which is love. So by finding out where that feeling died and bringing it back to life (assuming it was there in the first place), a person is able to plant the seed of God-Is-Love in the subconscious mind.

When God is viewed as a parent figure, Good Old Dad, then G.O.D. becomes an acronym. Many problems arise from this idea, which nourishes such beliefs as:

- God causes misery, punishment and trouble in the world.
- We are subservient and, therefore, not responsible for our circumstances.
- We must adhere to laws and beliefs that may conflict with what's in our best interest.

The Bible tells us at Genesis 1:26, "You are created in the image and likeness of God." Consequently, what we believe God to be is of utmost importance. Helen Street Paredes states it thusly:

> It is done unto you as you believe. If you believe in a judgmental God, you are judgmental and judged; if you believe in a loving God, you are loving and loved.[4]

From this vantage point, I work with my patients. Nearly 100 years after Freudian psychology separated the psychological and spiritual aspects of mental health, the New Age Movement and the Recovery Movement have now begun to reconcile these two halves of the human psyche. Medical hypnoanalysts have been doing this since Dr. Bryan began the treatment in 1955. J. Gordon Melton, Ph.D., Director of the Institute for the Study of American Religion and author of the *Encyclopedia of American Religions*, credits the New Thought with the "ability to empower people who feel, for whatever reason, that they are powerless."[5] He writes:

> New Thought has shown an amazing ability to speak to these people and teach them about their inner resources, to teach them what their own negative approaches and vision of the world is doing to them. By getting a more positive outlook on life, these people are developing a greater sense of their own worth and a greater sense of their own capabilities. They are empowered to make use of their inner talents and to turn sickness into health.[6]

Every Man Was a "Mister Right"

Cassie, 32, came in complaining that she experienced trouble verbalizing her thoughts, had a short memory, and got attached to people. Her self-image was low. She'd had therapy elsewhere and recognized her Ponce de Leon syndrome with spiritual overtones.

I asked what made it worse and she said, "If someone interrupts me or becomes forceful, or if I don't feel comfortable with someone, in crowds or social gatherings."

When I asked what made it better, she said, "When I have had my grief, been close, or even if I have had a good interaction, it restores my faith."

Both of those responses sounded like what would be heard from a scared kid, so I asked what she would be able to do once she was cured that she couldn't do now. She said, "Leave home, start to take care of myself, feel confident, have relationships."

Grow up, in other words. Other things in her history pointed to a Ponce de Leon diagnosis. Cassie was standing in the fountain of youth outside the stream of life. She said that she had never had an affair, that she scared men away because she treated everybody she went to bed with as a potential "Mr. Right."

The attitude that every man was a potential Mr. Right indicated an underlying addictive need for love and comfort that was not getting fulfilled. Of course, that clinging, childlike behavior would drive men away.

Cassie was reared Catholic[7], and had developed feelings of personal guilt and inadequacy because of her behavior. Here are some of her responses to my questions during the history-taking period of our first session:

Ryan: What was traumatic for you?

Cassie: My mother. She always escalated. I was very much afraid of her. (She looked up to heaven.) I think I was sexually abused. Also, I just recently had a relationship and it was scary.

Ryan: When you were school-age, did you sleepwalk or have nightmares.

Cassie: I sleepwalked, but I also would cry on the way to school. I didn't feel connected and wanted to stay home.

Ryan: Did you have repeated or recurring dreams?

Cassie: I often dreamed that there was a gloved hand under the bed trying to grab me.

Ryan: Tell me about your childhood.

Cassie: I was angry and depressed.

Ryan: Tell me about your parents.

Cassie: They were constantly fighting.

Ryan: What do you feel most guilty about in your life?

Cassie: I used to feel guilty about masturbating.

Ryan: What's the worst thing that happened to you?

Cassie: It's my mother. She destroys me verbally.

RYAN: Is there anything you haven't told me that I should know?

CASSIE: When I was in the city, I was pretty promiscuous. And I used to do a lot of drugs.

RYAN: What do you want from me?

CASSIE: I don't want to feel strange about sex, I want not to be afraid of bitchy, dominating women, and I want to plan my future so I'll have a good job.

Cassie's responses indicated some spiritual concerns in addition to the Ponce de Leon tendencies. People who behave promiscuously, do drugs, and also drink frequently are, among other things, trying to make themselves feel more alive.

Under hypnosis, I regressed Cassie to the time when she experienced sexual abuse from her mother.[8] She was about nine months old. It took several sessions to work through this experience. After relieving the anxiety, fear, and anger and being able to associate the problems she had in relationships in the here and now with that frightful experience when she was small, we were able to help her free up her subconscious and grow up and no longer be afraid of relationships and of other people. Both she and I thought she was cured.

A year later, she came in with another problem. Here is our conversation:

RYAN: What's the problem?

CASSIE: It's peer-related. (Then she looked up to heaven.) Just that. I'll stick to that. Being accepted by a group. I feel like a tag-a-long. I can't compete in conversation. I get scared, clam up, and feel inadequate. I am a pleaser. To make up for other people's lack of interest in me, I get needy. That is part of the problem with the relationship I was in. I was putting all this energy into other people, thinking they would come back, and they wouldn't. I would have to stand on my head to get what I wanted—attention and recognition.

RYAN: How long has it been a problem?

CASSIE: All my life. It was very troublesome when I was in high school. I was a lost puppy. My whole family was against me. I never felt adequate. It comes up again and again.

RYAN: What conditions cause variations in the problem?

CASSIE: It's generally the voice in my head; the scary critical voice.

RYAN: What makes it better?

CASSIE: Attention from my boyfriend.

Ryan: What will you be able to do once you are cured that you cannot do now?

Cassie: (She looked up to heaven.) Feel confident with myself, have lasting relationships, consistent friendships and a strong sense of self.

Once again, we worked through her childhood trauma, her use of drugs, her guilt feelings, and ways she was punishing herself. I did two prenatal regressions and helped her recognize her mother's negative attitude about the pregnancy. She was able to accept that those feelings belonged to her mother, not to her, and identified some of her own early feelings of peace and confidence that she could bring back to the present. I suggested that she increase her feeling of being connected to God and the universe and helped her to identify with nature and feel like she belonged in the world. Getting to the initial sensitizing event—in the womb at three months when she felt unwanted—provided the solution to Cassie's problem. Her story has a very happy ending.

Once we relieved the anxiety causing her underlying identity problem, she was quickly able to mend the hole in her spirit. She began to feel connected and was able to finish her education. She even got an advanced degree. She met someone and they fell in love. The last contact I had with her she was happily married and looking forward to the birth of her second child.

Cassie had finally been able to overcome a lifetime of spiritual illness and recover her spiritual health. Spiritual walking-zombie problems such as Cassie's, as you'll remember, frequently begin in the womb and often indicate a lack of connection with "God" and to the universe. After all, to a fetus or child, who, if not mother, is God?

MENTAL HEALTH REQUIRES "BEING RIGHT WITH GOD"

History shows us that "being right with God" has always been a precondition for physical and mental health. Before the advent of medical research, the absence of health was considered only a spiritual matter, to be rectified through spiritual practices, faith healing, laying on of hands, praying, casting out demons, oils, rituals, and sacrifices. The source of many of the guilt feelings and emotional disorders I find in patients can be traced back to misinformation and distortions that were received before the patient was able to discern negative suggestions.

Thanks to Dr. Bryan's contributions, therapists and clients alike can benefit from a mind-body-spirit union concept. Being a very spiritual man, Dr. Bryan melded his knowledge of law, psychology, and medicine with religion to produce a consistent and practical approach to psychospiritual health.

The Bible tells us that much of our anxiety amounts to a denial of God, which is a denial of peace and love and an acceptance of guilt. We deny ourselves peace and love when we indulge in judging ourselves and others, resulting in guilt and self-punishment.

Bryan went back to the original Biblical passages to define a person's relationship to God—to find what was required to be right with one's Maker. Likewise, people experiencing the psychological effects of guilt need to reexamine the source of those feelings, and the best way to get back to the source of guilt-producing events in our lives is through subconscious analysis to locate the time and place at which the negative thought was accepted.

Bryan reminded us that humans, once created, were given responsibility for their own lives:

> So God created man in his own image, in the image of God he created him; male and female he created them. God blessed them and said to them, "Be fruitful and increase in number; fill the earth and subdue it. Rule over the fish of the sea and the birds of the air and over every living creature that moves on the ground.[9]

In seeking to combat people's attitudes about guilt, he also examined the apostle Paul's interpretation of Christians' frequent guilt response to breaking the Ten Commandments in light of the purpose of Christ's act of atonement. Paul, who was also a lawyer, explains in his letter to the Galatians that adherence to the Jewish law cannot justify any person, but that faith in Jesus Christ is what saves them.

> We . . . know that a man is not justified by observing the law, but by faith in Jesus Christ. So we, too, have put our faith in Christ Jesus that we may be justified by faith in Christ and not by observing the law, because by observing the law, no one will be justified.[10]

> I do not set aside the grace of God, for if righteousness could be gained through the law, Christ died for nothing![11]

Paul then explains that God made a promise to Abraham:

> . . . He believed God, and it was credited to him as righteousness.[12]

In the same chapter, Bryan notes that Paul, in writing to the Galatian congregations, invalidates the claim that the Ten Commandments have anything to do with salvation and, therefore, with guilt:

> The promises were spoken to Abraham and to his seed. The Scripture does not say 'and to seeds,' meaning many people, but 'and to your seed,' meaning one person, who is Christ. What I mean is this: The law, introduced 430 years later, does not set aside the covenant previously established by God and thus do away with the promise. For if the inheritance depends on the law, then it no longer depends on a promise; but God in his grace gave it to Abraham through a promise.[13]

In the paragraph preceding this selection, Paul wrote that Christ had brought us out from the doom of that impossible system, meaning strict compliance with the law. Consequently, people today who feel depressed about their lack of righteousness under the rules and regulations of the Ten Commandments are judging themselves by a standard that doesn't apply. Since Christ's death, the commandments are null and void. They do not count. Well, then you may be thinking, why are they there? Paul explains:

> What, then, was the purpose of the law? It was added because of transgressions until the Seed to whom the promise referred had come. . . .
>
> Is the law, therefore, opposed to the promises of God? Absolutely not! For if a law had been given that could impart life, then righteousness would have come by the law. But the Scripture declares that the whole world is a prisoner of sin, so that what was promised, being given through *faith in Jesus Christ*, might be *given to those who believe*.[14] [Italics mine.]

Paul then asks in chapter 3 verse 21 if God is confused, first making promises and then contradicting himself with laws. "Of course not," he says. And, at the end of this chapter, he sums up the whole matter by claiming that we were in **protective custody** by the law until Christ arrived, who thereupon freed us from the bondage to law, freed us to be heirs to God's promise as descendents of Abraham—through faith and belief in Jesus Christ.

> Before this faith came, we were held prisoners by the law, locked in until faith should be revealed. So the law was put in charge to lead us to Christ that we might be justified by faith. Now that faith has come, we are no longer under the supervision of the law. . . . If you belong to Christ, then you are Abraham's seed, and heirs according to the promise.[15]

And, that is that. An act of faith, not strict compliance with the law, merits salvation. Guilt is neither virtuous nor desirable in the eyes of God. The commandments are not our means of salvation.

Instead of internalizing guilt, depressing our spirits and compounding our emotional problems as a result of our behavior, it is more appropriate that we ask who gave us the right to punish ourselves? Or even to judge ourselves? Isn't that God's job? Didn't God send Jesus to atone for all the sins committed by all the people who ever lived or ever will live? And isn't that forgiveness available for the asking? Yes! So it follows that judging ourselves is usurping God's jurisdiction. It's like telling God that he didn't do enough by sending Jesus. He should have done more! Maybe a sequel is necessary—Jesus II.

GUILT CARRIES FROM LIFETIME TO LIFETIME

Often, guilt and depression stem from incidents that took place in a personal history, long forgotten and subconsciously activated. When a person comes to my office suffering from depression, I use hypnosis to analyze the subconscious mind, to identify the negative suggestion, and determine when the suggestion was taken in. In other words, I search out the initial sensitizing event. This locating process involves age regressions and sometimes past-life regressions, either spontaneously or directed by request. Guilt carries on from lifetime to lifetime.

Frequently, depressed people who seek past-life therapy are consciously convinced they've been taken advantage of or mistreated. I've found in regressions that usually people will go first to lifetimes where they were victimized, where they were murdered or raped, for example. The natural tendency is to return to traumatic experiences that left them with fear. It may take several regressions before patients go to lives during which they were perpetrators of evil or wrongdoing, where they hurt others. But that is where the guilt lies.

The value of past-life therapy is that, through viewing several lifetimes, those who believe expand awareness of the permanency of the soul, which helps in spiritual development.[16] I was a female in some incarnations, a Spaniard, an Atlantean, a farmer, a pirate, an Eastern Indian, and a Native American. Many of my earlier lives have been negative. It was very difficult and humbling, for instance, to review myself slaying my decrepit mother. In this life, I feel I am serving, therefore, making a positive impact.

Guilt across the Ages

Kitty came to me bearing a burden of guilt. She called it Catholic guilt—she had been brought up in a strict Catholic environment. She had plenty of guilt, but she didn't know why.

Our search for an answer led us back to an incident that happened when she was 17. Kitty had got drunk and had sex with two guys. Now she was middle-aged and the guilt still clung.

We explored the here and now through age regression and found nothing to explain her present feelings. Then we began exploring past lives, and the ISE surfaced.

Kitty's subconscious mind held memories of a life several centuries in the past. As a young girl, she had romanced two young men simultaneously. She had married one while carrying the other's child. She never told her husband that the child she bore was fathered by another lover, and the guilt from that deception followed her into her present life.

Once we had identified the source of her guilt, Kitty was able to let it go. She began living the life she wanted to lead, unshackled by the guilt her subconscious harbored over an indiscretion subconsciously remembered from another life centuries before.

The Baby and the Bath Water

Most of the time it's unnecessary to regress to a previous existence. Many spiritual problems stem from long-forgotten experiences in our present life—long forgotten, that is, to our conscious minds.

Martin was a friend of mine, and in the course of our friendship he told me his problem. He was unable to get close to the opposite sex. When he tried to get close to women, he felt smothered.

Martin began treatment with a fellow analyst and was regressed to the first year of his life. His subconscious took him in memory to a scene in which he was in the bathtub and his mother was apparently stimulating his penis. His father walked in and threw a fit. During the argument, his mother started taking it out on the infant by holding his head under water.

During the regression, Martin described the sheer terror he felt at being helplessly submerged by his mother. And that's how he felt in his relationships with women as an adult. His subconscious was returning him to that feeling of having his head under water.

Hypnoanalysis helped Martin eject that feeling from his subconscious mind. With repetition and reinforcement of positive suggestions, he was free to enjoy his associations with women. Martin began dating after this point in treatment.

Martin had been experiencing a death suggestion on all levels. On the spiritual level, he felt that he had been rejected. On the physical level, he felt as if he were dying. That incident in the bathtub was the beginning of his problem with self-esteem, and it set him up for problems with women as well as for problems in other areas.

ARE YOU ALREADY DEAD?

"Most people die around 55 and are buried very much later," George Bernard Shaw said. That thought is worth considering as we examine faith and spirituality and their impact on mental health.

People with mature faith are curious. They are alert and looking ahead. They're excited about life. When people become static, when they don't ask questions and are willing to settle for existing conditions rather than seeking an abundant life, or when they become depressed and negative, they turn into spiritual walking zombies. It's time to search for causes, ask questions, and probe into events earlier in their existence. Medical hypnoanalysis is the best vehicle through which to conduct the search. The hypnoanalytic approach that has grown out of Bryan's work can best be described as psychospiritual. The psychopathology of spiritual walking zombies is that they have already accepted the suggestion that they are dead spiritually.

Max Was a Zombie

Max came to my office with a spiritual problem masking as sexual dysfunction. I record my clients' exact words to help in reaching a diagnosis. When I asked Max, "What's the problem?" he responded:

> Okay, well, I enjoyed listening to you speak the other day. It struck a chord as you being a person who could help me with my problems relating to circumcision. I was circumcised when I was born. It's a barbaric practice. I had something done to me. For one thing, I am gay. I'm in tune with the male's body. I like the uncircumcised penis. It's very difficult to find sexual partners who are uncircumcised.

When I asked how long this had been a problem, he said, "Well, I have been aware of it almost all my life. It's been more of a problem the last 10 to 15 years."

I asked what makes the problem worse and he said, "Nothing that I can think of. If I start reading some of the books I have."

To the question, "What makes it better?" He responded, "Finding a man who has a nice foreskin."

Then—and this is the important part—I said, "What will you be able to do once you're cured that you can't do now?"

He said, "Well," and he looked up to heaven and continued, "I guess something I've noticed, if one focuses on lack then one has a lack in their life. It stops me from really enjoying who I am right now. That anger and resentment comes up, stops me from enjoying other men completely who are cut."

Max, 35, had been focusing on his lack and that was the bottom line on where his problem lay. His focusing on his penis was only a symptom of the problem.

I asked about siblings. He had two brothers and a sister and commented that he went through a time thinking that his parents wanted a girl instead of him. About his childhood, he commented that, off and on, he had some unhappy times and did not always, or often, get along with his father. Concerned about Max's attitude, his parents had sent him to a psychologist when he was between 8 and 10 years of age.

In talking about problems surrounding his birth, he said he was born a month early and spent five or six days in an incubator.

> The doctor held me and said, "If he'll eat, he'll be okay."

I asked Max what he wanted from me, and he said he wanted to feel more relaxed about being circumcised. Then, he looked up to heaven again and said, "Just to get over the feeling of lack."

I felt I was on the right trail in the word-association test.

Ryan: Death . . .
Max: Life.
Ryan: Live . . .
Max: Life.
Ryan: Birth . . .
Max: Death.

So I could conclude that life was somehow connected in his subconscious mind with death, and the connection was coming from birth. Not only that, this fellow was gay and that had to be considered in his responses.

RYAN: Exciting . . .
MAX: Men.
RYAN: Depressed . . .
MAX: Excited.

Remember the rule of logic that applies in our word-association tests: If A=B and B=C, then A=C. So excited, depressed, and men all equal each other in Max's mind. That has a connection, subconsciously, to his feelings about himself and other men.

RYAN: This is where the problem came out . . .
MAX: A girl.
RYAN: Complete a sentence with the word "why."
MAX: Why am I here?

That was an indication that he had an identity problem, the fact that he thought his parents really wanted a girl.

RYAN: When did it start?
MAX: When I was born.
RYAN: Punishment.
MAX: I punish myself when I don't succeed. My punishment is denying myself.

He also brought up that he was not really doing the kind of work he wanted to do. We reviewed his history and word-association test, and he understood that he had an identity problem, that he felt unwanted and was a spiritual walking zombie because he was punishing himself.

THE DREAM

As with all my patients, I requested that Max bring in a dream. His was short and reflected both his dissatisfaction with his job and his homosexuality. He said, "The boss kept wanting this one cowboy type in tight blue jeans, with a cute butt, to talk about the weather on the news. I kept avoiding him. Finally, I acquiesced and got the interview."

Max said that after he wrote the dream down he forgot what it meant to him. "I sort of felt, at the time, like I feel in my life—like I am an observer and lonely." While he was under hypnosis, I asked him to go back to a time when he first felt that way, and he described a childhood scene in the family kitchen:

> My dad's up on a ladder. I'm on the floor. It's after my teacher told my mother I was lying. He yelled at me. He wouldn't believe me. I felt angry. I cried. I begged and I pleaded. I shut off and said, "I am not going to tell anything to anybody, ever." It mattered because I was right. I wanted him to believe me and to be loved by him.

We discussed that his decision, based on that one particular situation with his father, was in essence to go dead in his feelings. This was typical of what was happening in his life. He would cut his feelings off and go completely dead. I asked him to bring himself back to life, which he agreed to do. In a subsequent session, I regressed him to the womb and got this response:

> I feel tense, I felt tense all the way to today's experience. I'm scared, at five months. Maybe she's afraid that there isn't enough money, I don't know. It's just too cold. I don't have enough to pay the bills.

Max described feeling cold now when he doesn't have enough to pay the bills. It was significant that he identified these feelings both in the here and now and as belonging to his mother, since he did not have the ability to think separately and independently while he was in the womb.

The next step was to bring him through the birth experience, from five months to nine months intrauterine. During the experience, he said:

> Sometimes, I get this feeling the world is on top of me and I'm just squooshed.

He went through a good deal of physical discomfort and was wiggling around on the chair and crying slightly, so we wiped out what is called the "birth trauma." I also wiped out, removed from his subconscious, the "weight of the world," so he wouldn't have to carry it around. We removed the negative suggestion that was focused on his foreskin as a symbol of something he lacked. I gave him positive suggestions about being peaceful and calm and getting rid of the thoughts that his mother had about him, about feeling like he was supposed to be a girl, and about not belonging in the world.

Max came for a total of 14 sessions, three more after the womb regression, and each of those last three times said he was feeling better, more peaceful, and that his work was good. Once we removed the negative suggestions and he was able to feel loving towards himself, or God's love, he was cured. He changed jobs and the circumcised foreskin was a forgotten issue.

LET'S TAKE A HOLISTIC VIEW

Each individual is a combination of body, mind, and spirit. If any aspect is neglected, the person is in trouble. We each have the power to shape and control our destinies. Faith is the tool with which we try to understand our being and our place in an ever-changing world. Faith is a human activity, not a thing we possess. It is part of our being.

"Confession is good for the soul" is more than a cliche. Holding negative feelings inside does, indeed, kill one's spirit, but it also affects the body. In his research on body image among women with eating disorders, Dr. James Pennebaker, a Southern Methodist University professor, concluded that confession of a burdensome secret resulted in dramatic physical effects.[17]

Pennebaker found that women who have undergone sexual trauma before 17 years of age are more prone than others to develop medical problems later in life. He concluded that this phenomenon arises from the shame and guilt these women usually associate with the events. The negative feelings prevent them from discussing their ordeals with anyone. They are unable to let go of something that needs to be cleansed.

Pennebaker followed that finding with laboratory studies to measure the immediate effect that confiding heavy secrets had on the body and learned that when volunteers disclosed a secret, their blood pressure and heart rate dropped and their sweat reflexes diminished.

FAITH'S POWER IS AMAZING

Studies have shown that patients who believe in their doctors do better after surgery than those without faith. They need less pain medication and have shorter hospital stays. Even ignoring the recorded incidents of people "thinking" themselves well, we have to admit that faith is intricately related to healing and that our bodies have a built-in healing system.

Faith is not religion, although religion is often the result of faith. People can be religious without faith. They are caught up in the rituals of religion.

Faith gives meaning to our lives. It means we don't fully understand, that we are acting on something we don't know.

The classic faith story involves a tightrope walker who strung his rope across the American side of Niagara Falls during the 1930s and crossed it pushing a wheelbarrow. When a crowd gathered to watch the spectacle, the artist asked, "How many believe I can do it again?" They all nodded in support, but when he called for a volunteer with enough faith to ride the wheelbarrow across the chasm, only a child whose parents were not present stepped forward.

The opposite of faith is worry. A lack of faith can lead to narcissism (worry about oneself), anxiety (worry about all sorts of things), or embittered pessimism (the belief that everything will turn out wrong). Happiness is a by-product of faith.

Dr. Thomas A. Ritzman wrote, and I concur:

> Religion is only one person's path to understanding God, and it may be very different from another's. The trouble comes when we try to force one religion upon somebody who thinks he has a better one, and it doesn't really make any difference what religion he has as long as it leads to the same place.
>
> God is creative energy. That we experience this energy as love; that within us it promotes order, happiness, life-energy, and all other things that we feel as 'good'; that we can receive this energy from those close to us and pass it on to others, is simple enough and easy to discuss consciously with depressed people or those with behavior problems resulting from depression.
>
> It helps to prepare the way for getting the concept of God as a judgment-day monster out of the minds of those with jurisdictional problems.[18]

Silver Needed to Mend His Connection with God

Silver's case was unusual. A 30-year-old male medical student with acute myologenous leukemia, he had heard me speak on subconsciously accepting and acting out death suggestions. Since his illness was not responding to traditional medical treatment and his medical doctors threw up their hands and gave him up for dead, he had decided to follow up on the possibility that he was subconsciously trying to cause his own death.

When I asked my usual, "What's the problem?" Silver responded:

> Acute myologenous leukemia. Or that may be the symptom of the problem. Fatigue. Bleeding from the nose, gums. Susceptibility to many infections.

I asked how long he had had the problem. He said, "Two years."

He had a life-threatening illness, and I already sensed he was subconsciously giving up his existence to maintain something of more importance to himself. My goal was to find what that important something was.

Without my prompting, he picked back up on his response to my "What's the problem?" saying:

> I am out of remission and they tell me that time is running out. Right now, I am having supportive treatment.

He also mentioned that he had two years of treatment in another state. He had recently gone to a mind-programming seminar and was interested in exploring what the power of the mind could do in his case.

When I asked him what he would be able to do once he was cured that he couldn't do now, he said:

> Well, my goals are to start a family. I have been married a year and a half. And I am not sure of my choice in the medical profession. (He was a resident.)

The number "two" and personal guilt kept coming up in the history-taking portion of the visit:

- He said he had **two** years of treatment.
- **Two** days after his supportive treatment he was back at home.
- On a scale of zero to ten, his life now was a one or **two**.
- He said he had completed close to **two** years of residency.
- He drank a beer or **two** every **couple** of days.
- I asked him about suicide and he looked up to heaven and said, "When I thought about it, it was pretty fleeting—a minute or **two**."
- He talked about a **two**-year age difference between him and his brother.
- I asked if his parents had ever been really concerned about him. He said, "**Twice**. I had an eye injury in fourth grade, and now."
- There was some heavy petting with a cousin about **two** years ago. (This information combined the number two and guilt feelings, since he was reared in a very strict orthodox religion.)

The last history question also provided useful information. I asked what he wanted from me, and he said:

> See if there is something in my past that is causing me to want to kill myself if, indeed, that is what I am doing. Also, another thing, my brother brought up low self-esteem. I've been an overachiever all my life.

Silver had thrown out several points that caught my attention, and I pursued them under hypnosis in a word-association test:

RYAN: I would rather die than . . .
SILVER: Be unhappy.
RYAN: The unhappiness began when . . .
SILVER: I started medical school.
RYAN: All my life . . .
SILVER: Work.

So all his life, Silver had been overworking to achieve. Through further word associations, it became clear that fear, worry, security, anxiety, self-esteem, death, and life were associated in his subconscious mind; that guilt equaled bad; that punishment equaled discipline; and that discipline equaled death. His life, therefore, was primarily focused on fear, anxiety, and death.

Silver had no self-love and was punishing himself. He was a spiritual walking zombie. Why? With Silver still under hypnosis, I continued the word-association test:

RYAN: I hate myself because . . .
SILVER: I am causing pain to others.
RYAN: Pain . . .
SILVER: Disease.
RYAN: Leukemia feels like . . .
SILVER: Pain.

He evidently felt guilty because, through his illness, he was causing other people to suffer.

RYAN: It all started when . . .
SILVER: I went to school.
RYAN: It got worse when . . .
SILVER: I wanted to get married.

Remember, this was done under hypnosis. These responses were coming from his subconscious mind.

Ryan: They really wanted . . .
Silver: A puppet.
Ryan: The person I would most like to make happy is . . .
Silver: Dad.
Ryan: Dad really wants . . .
Silver: A success.

Through the word-association test, we obtained a sketchy outline of what was happening in Silver's subconscious mind: He was punishing himself for some kind of problem. He felt his parents wanted a puppet. For a long time, he had been overachieving, trying to please them. He was unhappy with himself for doing that. The unhappiness began when he started medical school. And he would rather die than be unhappy. The picture that came from his subconscious, then, was of a person who was indirectly killing himself.

Silver's Dream Supports the Word-association Test Results

Silver's dream was set in the medical center:

> There were three offices in a row in a hospital. These offices were between two parallel hallways; hence, each had two doors: the main entrance off the main hallway, and the secondary entrance off a smaller hallway on the other side.
>
> I had the office on one end. The middle office was empty. Dr. Miguel (supervising physician in the residency program) had the office on the other end.
>
> I opened the secondary exit door, not knowing where it led to, and found myself in a large, luxury-type hangout with kitchen and entertainment facilities. Dr. Miguel greeted me and took me on tour. He made it known that I was privy to this set up, but was to keep it secret from the other residents as it was a special place for a select few.
>
> At this time, two girls sneaked into the secondary hallway and into the hangout. I slammed the door shut, but they kicked a hole through it. I replaced the door quickly and kept them out, then I forced them back down the hall and into my office.

> Through the back hall, I found more people, friends, in my office wanting to come into the hangout. I left them there, went back to the hangout to check it out. Found a bathroom. Had to urinate and did so.

When asked to interpret his dream, Silver said, "I was finally led into the inner group. It was good, but I was also worried about keeping everyone else out."

He related the dream to his college years and said the two girls represented his mother and his aunt. They would not accept his girlfriend then and he was angry about it. He had a lot of resentment bottled up inside.

Silver was intelligent and very good at analysis. He realized that the resentment was part of what was eating away at him, and, under hypnosis, agreed to stop sacrificing his feelings and his physical self for the approval of his mother and aunt. He had described how both of them had controlling personalities and how they dominated and overwhelmed him.

I felt that this part of the treatment went fairly well, but I was frustrated by the results of the regressions. It was very hard for this client to regress. I felt sure some early experience or situation had contributed to that problem, but I was reserving my judgment. This case was a challenge to me. Silver was extremely motivated to get better, and since he had a life-threatening disease, I very much wanted to help create a mind-set for healing his leukemia.

After discussing the dream, I talked to him about leukemia being a cancer of immature cells and, in a transcendental kind of association, connected it to the Ponce de Leon syndrome. He picked up on that and said that the parental pressure relented after he got sick.

The situation began to make more sense: His subconscious had developed an extremely rare, life-threatening sickness. A secondary gain from his illness was that by staying sick he was keeping his parents off his back.

That satisfied the primary subconscious analysis in the word-association test: He would rather be dead than cause others pain. It also satisfied the secondary proposition: keeping his parents from pressuring him to get well and to be a doctor, things he wasn't sure he wanted to do.

He experienced subconscious resistance during regression attempts, however. Regressed to seven months in the womb, he spoke of a problem, pain, and probably fear. Then, he stopped reporting and resisted any communication.

So, I tried regressing him back to the first time he felt he was killing himself off. He said:

> It's all jumbled up. There are flowers. Nowhere. Black. Nothing, really. All of these jumbled words in my head, but I can't make them out.

I interrupted suddenly and asked him to go back to the womb:

> A lot of pain. Anger. Maybe Dad is hitting Mom. She is crying. Me. 'Cause I am there! Cause Mom is sick. Mom is too sick to cook!

I interrupted again and asked him to move up to the birth. He did not; just said he wasn't feeling anything and resisted further. He did say that he understood Dad was hitting Mom because he, Silver, was there and that he was responsible for his mother's pain.

By tying that reaction to the word-association response that he would rather be dead than cause pain, I concluded that this was probably the initial sensitizing event for his decision to kill himself off. I removed that negative suggestion and the responsibility for believing that he caused his mother to get hit. He accepted my interpretations and felt relieved and very curious about these memories.

In a subsequent session, we talked about his recurring fears that he was not getting any better. At the first sign of his blood count changing negatively, he would become frightened and depressed. I explained that he was interfering with his self-healing abilities by negatively programming his subconscious mind with fear.

Silver's Childhood Regressions Were Productive

We discovered several death suggestions through regressions to Silver's childhood. One was a time when he almost lost an eye. We talked about times when he felt victimized and felt sorry for himself. We went to a time when he was beaten up as a child and noted how he internalized his anger. We went to a time when his grandmother had shouted, "If you children don't behave, I'll poke my eyes out." The child in Silver took that to heart, thinking he was hurting her by rebelling. He agreed to take responsibility for and express his feelings, especially anger.

Working with Silver was emotionally involving. His blood counts would change almost weekly. He was in and out of the hospital. It was nip and tuck. I grew attached to him. His battle became my battle.

We worked on his extreme desire, even willingness to sacrifice himself, to get his parents' approval. That factor weighed heavily on his mind.

One time I wanted to find out at what age his subconscious mind was operating and had him do an imagery in which he was in a movie theater. The theater lit up with, instead of a picture, the number 12, the age of the child within him. I regressed him to that age. He was in sixth grade, fat, not very popular in school, and experiencing fear of losing his mother. We identified that fear as a feeling still influencing him in the here and now. His mother's and aunt's dislike of his wife was forcing him to choose between them and again making him feel he was losing his mother. Consequently, he had subconsciously decided that he could satisfy his need to please everybody, keep the family together, get the attention he desired, and fulfill his need to be himself by dying.

I did as much as I could to remove his negative thought and behavior patterns. I removed the initial sensitizing event and several symptom-producing and symptom-intensifying events. Through this process, Silver developed a good understanding of himself and his relationship with God and with various family members. He was able to take charge of his feelings and thinking.

When I last talked with him, he was still fighting the leukemia, but with a different attitude. He had decided that it was up to him and God at that point, and he terminated treatment. He still had ups and downs that were beyond the comprehension of the medical profession but had developed a stronger faith and was working on healing himself through mental imagery and positive suggestions. Silver, his wife, and his brother all expressed the belief that his hypnoanalysis and his strong new-found connection to God had played the crucial role in his self-healing.

One day, after the first draft of this book had been written, Silver's brother called to tell me that Silver had died. The brother told me that I should know that both he and Silver felt that the treatment had bought the patient two years of life that he wouldn't have had otherwise.

I was extremely sad to know about his death, but it brought to mind something that Dr. Bryan said—a comment I think about when I've done everything I can for a patient—"Leave something to God."

WE ARE THE EXPERIMENT

Science is now recognizing a basis for what mystics, some religions, and metaphysical people have been saying for a long time: We are what we think. We affect our lives and the lives of others in ways we don't fully understand. We are the experiment. We are evolution in process, and we can affect our internal and external environments through the focus of our minds—our thoughts. When we change our minds, we change what will go on around us.

The television series "Quantum Leap," begun in the late 1980s, took its story line from this idea. In the show, a physics professor was caught in an earlier time warp and could not come up with the formula to get back to his present time and place. Weekly he found himself in the body of a different person who was facing a life crisis. Knowing the future, the physicist was able, through relationships and behavior, to influence history. A fanciful story? Not entirely. By our thoughts and actions, we do indeed control our piece of history.

God created each of us with a mind. It's unfortunate when we misuse it because of our failure to recognize its power. Yet, the subconscious mind is perhaps the most underutilized part of the mind, and much of what people do with it is to ignore it. Fear, depression, hate, failure, anxiety, deceit, self-doubt, and guilt are all negatives. Much of what we hear around us is negative. We can't change everything; however, we do have control over what we allow to get to our subconscious.

Since we're not perfect, we can't be proud of everything we do, but we can be proud of what we are. We are children of God—God's ultimate creation, in His image. If we cannot love ourselves first, we cannot love anybody else. So our experiment begins with programming love into our subconscious minds.

In response to a question from a learned man about the greatest commandment in the law, Jesus replied:

> Love the Lord your God with all your heart and with all your soul and with all your mind. This is the first and greatest commandment. And the second is like it: 'Love your neighbor as yourself.' All the Law and the Prophets hang on these two commandments.[19]

However, most people learn to love others better than themselves, which contradicts Jesus' message.

We develop personal power by balancing and directing our creative energies. Writer Elie Wiesel, a survivor of the holocaust, responds to the question "Why are we here?" in this way:

> Our obligation is to give meaning to life and in doing so to overcome the passive, indifferent life. A person who is indifferent is dead without knowing it. I believe that life has meaning in spite of the meaningless death I have seen. Death has no meaning, life has. We must make every minute rich and enriching, not for oneself, but for someone else, and thereby create a bridge between beings that limits the domain of nothingness. Life is a gift and meaning is its reward. The meaning of life is to be found in every encounter. Every moment is a moment of grace.[20]

We can make our lives different if we want to. We have the power to bring about change in ourselves and our environments through love, through devoting our mental energies to positive pursuits. There is an old Chinese proverb that says, "If you don't change your direction, you'll get exactly where you're heading."

God Is Not in Charge

Dana needed a change in direction when she came into my office suffering from depression and chronic substance abuse. She complained that her life had little meaning, that everything seemed void and empty, and that she "did not fit in."

> My depression and substance abuse were masking underlying problems which I refused to acknowledge. I had worked unsuccessfully with other counselors, but continued to block many emotional injuries and aspects of my upbringing in a dysfunctional family.
>
> I was spiritually empty and blamed God for allowing things I could not control to happen. Before I could change my attitude, I needed to acknowledge what it was, face those painful experiences and reprogram old belief systems.

Effective hypnoanalysis starts with identifying the thoughts and related reactions accepted at the time of the initial sensitizing event, and reinforced later, which are blocking acceptance and use of divine energy, i.e. love. After removal of these beliefs and thoughts, a new concept of self can be presented and reinforced.

Dana went on:

> I now realize that I have control over my own life and have accepted total responsibility. I have made and continue to make necessary changes in order to free myself from the curses of my childhood.
>
> The hypnoanalytic process has been extremely worthwhile for me. Now, I feel alive.

Dana was brought up in an abusive family with a mother who required her children to adopt the same fundamental Christian beliefs that she had. As a recourse to the fire-and-brimstone upbringing, backed by the fury of an ever-present switch, Dana began using drugs as a teenager. She continued her drug use through two marriages, even marrying a fellow who was a user much like herself. When she came for treatment, her problem was "sustained alcohol and drug abuse." Dana's treatment was intense, and more protracted than is my usual case. For all practical purposes, Dana's emotional and spiritual growth had ceased when she grew into puberty. Being well-motivated, she stopped the marijuana use and cut down on her alcohol consumption. Then, we worked on her identity problem and her immaturity. The following is her description of her problems once she stopped her substance abuse:

> When I have to talk about myself, I get real anxious and uncomfortable. I get worse when I have to discuss feelings.

When I asked her what she wanted, she said:

> To be true to myself; to be assertive; to honestly and openly state how I feel.

After five months of working on Dana's goals, I received this letter from her:

> Dear Ryan:
>
> A year and a half ago, I came to see you, a shell of a person burned out on life, probably not caring whether I ever saw another sunset or sunrise. The void I lived with was [there] because I had lost all faith and thus all hope in this seemingly cruel, lifeless existence, and felt helpless to do anything to ease the pain in a constructive way.
>
> But since then, there have been many changes. The most important has been the spiritual awakening that I have most recently begun exploring. This spiritual journey has become the most exciting venture I have ever experienced. Working on my past religious upbringing has freed me so that I may now learn and explore without feeling guilt and without displaced anger. Most recently, I do not live, act and feel like a spiritual zombie, but instead like a spiritual embryo—alive and growing.

This is what therapy is about for me. It fills a need I have to be involved in helping others as well as myself to learn to "love your neighbor AS YOURSELF." I added the capitals to emphasize what we all know instinctively: that love begins at home, with oneself.

"For I am convinced," wrote Dostoevski in *The Brothers Karamazov*, "that the only hell that exists is the inability to love." I would add "oneself, especially."

Dana "got it," so to speak. She was healed and helped due to the power of love, which is another word for God.

WE CAN DO IT

Remember, problems are mind over matter, to borrow from Mark Twain. If you don't mind, then they don't matter. Change has a cumulative effect. There is a divine principle operating inside each of us. We are all connected in some fundamental way, and when one person changes, it brings change in others.

You may know the story told in *The Hundredth Monkey*. According to Ken Keyes, who reported the phenomenon, one young monkey of a tribe in a remote setting started taking his food to the water's edge to wash the grit off before eating it. Other monkeys saw the action and gradually followed the young one's example. Monkeys at other locations were observed continuing to eat unwashed food, however. At the exact time that the hundredth monkey in the original colony began washing his food, the practice was begun by primates at other sites all over the world. Without being taught or observing the washing activity, the knowledge and practice had spread through the monkeys' collective intelligence.[21]

If enough of us devote our mental energies to removing our negativity and focusing on positive pursuits, we will, through our collective consciousness, bring about a better world. Belief is the key. If we believe we can make a better world, we can.

W. Clement Stone, Chicago philanthropist and CEO of the Combined Insurance Companies, is famous for having said, "Whatever the mind can conceive and believe it can achieve." One person's mind is a microcosm of the whole world. And who knows? You may be the one hundredth human, who turns the tide in the world.

Key Concepts

- What we feel in relation to our self-image and self-esteem results from how much God we have in our lives.
- In some 50 percent of the cases of depression, low self-esteem, or chronic guilt, and nearly all cases of addiction and abuse, the subconscious root of the problem refers to people's concept of God. Man has created God in man's image.
- History indicates that "being right with God" has always been a precondition for physical and mental health.
- Humans, once created, are given responsibility for their own lives. Life is for the creating.
- People today who feel depressed about their lack of righteousness under the Ten Commandments are judging themselves by a standard that no longer applies.
- Guilt is neither virtuous nor desirable in the eyes of God.
- The value of past-life therapy is that, through viewing several lifetimes, our awareness is greatly expanded and we can more clearly evaluate our lives and the primacy of the soul.
- Each individual is a combination of body, mind, and spirit. If any aspect is neglected, the person is in an unbalanced state. All areas need to be fed.
- We are evolution in process. When we change our minds, we change what will go on around us.
- We develop personal power by balancing and directing our creative energies.
- We are all connected in some fundamental way, and when one person changes, it brings change in others and to his or her environment.

Growth Exercise

1. State in a sentence or two what you think God is. What is God like?

2. Are you sure you want to hold on to that view of God?

3. How much does that view resemble someone important to you in an earlier life? Good Old Dad? Or Good Old Mom?

4. What transgressions do you feel guilt over? List them.

5. Point out the transgressions on this list that Jesus didn't die for.

6. How are you punishing yourself?

7. Do you intend to continue?

8. List 10 things you can do to put more love (God) in your life?

CHAPTER THIRTEEN

WIDE AWAKE, CLEAR HEADED, AND REFRESHED . . .

Good judgment comes from experience.
And where does experience come from?
Experience comes from bad judgment.

—*Mark Twain*

A FEW LAST WORDS

The title of this book and this last chapter is the last thing I say to a client as he or she comes out of the hypnotic state. Being consistent then, I believe it's best said last to you, the reader, because we are all in a trance, or we've all been in a trance of our own. If you've read this far, you've read about people who changed their trance, underwent transformation as well as learned about "trance"-formation. True freedom is the ability to change one's trance. The inability to change one's trance is neurosis.

The Roman Emperor Marcus Aurelius said it centuries ago, "If you are pained by external things, it is not they that disturb you, but your own judgement of them. And it is in your power to wipe out that judgement now." John Stuart Mill said it thusly, "No great improvements in the lot of mankind are possible until a great change takes place in the fundamental constitution of their modes of thought."

So, *Wide Awake, Clear Headed, and Refreshed* . . .to me means that happiness is in our own chosing once we wake up to the power of our minds, clear our heads of the baggage and negative suggestions and misinformation, and finally refresh our spirits with our God-given ability to create ourselves and our lives the way we desire.

The question then is how does one know what to create. The following passage gets to my point.

> The greatest margin of success is achieved by anyone doing what they want to do more than all other things . . . do what brings the greatest happiness, whatever it is. For when you are joyful, that creates the aura of abundance from the Divine Source. When you're happy, God the Father gives you everything you want. . . .
>
> —Ramtha the Enlightened One

APPENDIX A

METHODS OF SELF-HYPNOSIS

The self-hypnosis blackboard. This method is suggested by George Honiotes, M.D.:

> You want to enter a suggestion into your subconscious mind. The suggestion may be, "I'm going to wake up at 6 o'clock tomorrow," or "I'm going to slim down so I can wear the bathing suit I saw in the store window today," or "I'm going to cut a second off my best time in the 100-meter race." Once you have decided on the suggestion, find a good bed or sofa, and make yourself comfortable. Pick a spot on a wall or ceiling and stare at it. If you stare at anything long enough, you'll get tired of staring. When you reach that point, tell yourself that you are going to count from one to five, and at the count of five you will let your eyes close and will let yourself relax. Remember: You do not close your eyes and you do not relax yourself. You *let* your eyes close and you *let* yourself relax. After you let your eyes close, you let yourself begin to relax, and as you relax you imagine a blackboard with the numbers 50 to 0 written on it in iridescent chalk. In your imagination, you visualize the numbers, and you also visualize two or three key words from your desired suggestion, written in iridescent chalk at the top of the blackboard and above the numbers. In your imagination, you begin to erase these numbers, one at a time, from 50 down to 0. As you do, you imagine that those key words glow brighter and brighter, like neon signs. Each time you breathe, you erase a number, so that you take 50 breaths as you erase from 50 down to 0 and as the words from your suggestion glow brighter and brighter. You now have complete control of yourself. You are permitting yourself to do this for yourself, so that after you have all the numbers erased and have breathed 50 times, you say to yourself, "I will now count myself up to 3 and be wide awake and alert, refreshed, full of life

and relaxed." And you will. This exercise should be practiced regularly, at least twice a day every day.

The hypnotist in the mirror. This method is suggested by Thomas J. Hopwood:

> Imagine that you are a famous hypnotist. It could be someone you actually know of, but don't know personally. Or it could be someone from your imagination.
>
> Now put on a pair of slippers and get comfortable. Imagine how this hypnotist would hypnotize a person using the direct gaze technique. Stand before your mirror, looking at the reflection of light in one of your eyes.
>
> Now imagine that you're another person—someone about to undergo hypnosis by your imaginary hypnotist. You may name this person if you wish. Call her Pat. Or call him Pat. Remember, you are not going to hypnotize yourself. Your imaginary hypnotist is going to hypnotize Pat. You are simply a detached observer.
>
> Now let your hypnotist talk to Pat, using any well-known hypnotic pattern. Don't just think the words; speak them, and form them clearly with your lips. This imparts more feeling to the words than thought alone.
>
> As you speak, try to imagine yourself in the roles of Pat and the hypnotist, now one, now the other or, even better, both at once.
>
> If the eyes grow cloudy for a second, it means Pat is going under. If you find the eyes beginning to wander, it's the hypnotist checking the progress of the subject. Now focus the eyes back on the light reflection in the iris as the hypnotist proceeds. When you feel your body swaying slightly, it means, again, that Pat is going under. The hypnotist will hear any noise or distraction, but Pat pays very little attention to these, hearing only the rhythmic sounds. imagine that the hypnotist is now ready to bring Pat completely under. This has no effect on you, of course; you're a detached bystander.
>
> "I'm going to count from 10 to 1 very slowly," the hypnotist tells Pat, "and during this count your right arm will begin to rise so that by the count of one, it will be straight out from your side. Ten, your arm is slowly rising, just an inch or two from your side; nine, your arm is still rising, slowly, steadily, it forms a slender "A" with the rest of your body; eight. . . ." With each count the rising suggestion will be given, with variations.
>
> As the hypnotist counts, Pat will be imagining how it would feel if the right arm did begin to rise. While Pat is imagining, the arm may make some movement other than that of rising. It may, for instance, make a small circular movement. The hypnotist is unperturbed. "Seven, as it slowly rises, your arm is moving in small circles. . . ." When the count of 1 is reached, Pat's arm will be at right angles to the body. As a detached observer, you know that this was not entirely brought about by the

hypnotist's suggestions. The arm could have remained at the side as easily as it rose, but Pat was merely going along with the hypnotist to get the sensation of being hypnotized.

The hypnotist now tells Pat that the arm is becoming rigid. "It's becoming as stiff as a board. It will not bend. When I count from three to one, it will be so rigid that you will be unable to bend it." When the count of one is reached, the hypnotist challenges Pat to bend the arm. Pat finds the arm is not as easy to bend, and tries harder. The arm will not bend. The hypnotist now tells Pat to stop trying. "Your arm will become relaxed. . . ."

The hypnotist may now deepen the trance, by a count, or by suggestions, or in some other way. Pat will be reminded that background noises will be audible, but attention should be focused on the hypnotist's voice. The hypnotist may now tell Pat to resume some relaxed position, and may give any suggestion deemed desirable. He will suggest that the next time Pat is hypnotized, a deeper and quicker hypnotic state will be attained.

In this exercise, you are not trying to hypnotize yourself. You're merely trying to imagine the feelings of hypnotist and subject. And you weren't hypnotized. Were you?

APPENDIX B

HOW TO TELL IF YOU WERE HYPNOTIZED

When you awake from sleep, you usually know you've been asleep; you are aware of the return of consciousness. But hypnosis is not sleep. While under hypnosis, you're aware of the things happening around you. You're relaxed, but your mind is concentrated. There is no "waking" in the sense of a return to consciousness. How, then, can you know when you've been hypnotized?

There are a number of signs.

Under hypnosis, you may feel numb or tingling, light or heavy. Your eyes may water and your eyelids may flutter. Your saliva glands may go into overproduction, causing you to swallow frequently.

You may have a feeling of daydreaming, of floating, of detachment.

As the hypnotist gives his suggestions, you may have thought to yourself: "I didn't have to follow the suggestions; I just felt like it. I could have resisted, but it was so easy to go along with it." Under hypnosis, there is no carrying out the suggestions because you *had* to obey. You may act on the suggestions out of a compelling desire to do so. You may even carry out the suggestion without knowing it.

As you're entering hypnosis, there will be an extreme concentration on the hypnotist's voice. If you hear other sounds, they will not bother you. They may be faint or beyond your awareness. To you, the only pertinent sound is that of the hypnotist's voice.

Under hypnosis, you will be superaware. You may hear clearly sounds or voices that you were unaware of in the normal state.

You may experience a strong belief that you can carry out the suggestions, from the hypnotist or from yourself, or that you can reach your goal. That feeling will remain after you have returned to the normal state.

You may lose track of conscious time. Twenty minutes may seem like five minutes. You may or may not remember everything or anything that happened while you were under hypnosis.

You may achieve a state of such relaxation that you didn't feel like opening your eyes on command and may even have resented the suggestion. You may have tried to open your eyes before the command but found that you couldn't.

Sometimes, people under hypnosis may be in an uncomfortable position, may have an itch or an urge to swallow cough or sneeze. They will do nothing about it because it requires too much effort.

You may experience things that don't normally occur. For example, you may be unaware of your body.

All these phenomena are indications that you experienced hypnosis, but they are not always present during hypnosis. The true test is whether you are making progress toward the goal you've set for yourself. By picking a certain time, giving yourself the same or similar suggestions and doing so for 30 days, you should find a change in yourself.

Let me know what happens by writing to:

Ryan Elliott
P.O. Box 535
Winfield, IL 60190

APPENDIX C

AMERICAN ACADEMY OF MEDICAL HYPNOANALYSTS

The American Academy of Medical Hypnoanalysts is an organization of professional psychotherapists who specialize in the practice of medical hypnoanalysis in that the preponderance of their work is spent in the practice of this modality.

The A.A.M.H., which was founded in May of 1974, is a non-profit organization dedicated to fostering and stimulating interest in Medical Hypnoanalysis. The Academy encourages and promotes research and education in hypnosis and hypnoanalysis; as well as propagating the practice of medical hypnoanalysis as a specialty. It provides interaction with colleagues, fosters professional stimulation, and improvement of services and knowledge of the modality to the public. It is dedicated to improving the care of patients/clients and promoting integrated well-being on mental, physical, emotional and spirituals levels.

It is the practice of the Academy to meet semi-annually with seminars on designated subjects.

The A.A.M.H. sponsors a periodical, *Medical Hypnoanalysis Journal,* which is published quarterly. This journal focuses on practical articles and serves as a forum for publication of research, new concepts and therapeutic tape scripts.

Membership

Professionals in mental health, psychological, medical and/or counseling fields with a Masters or higher qualify for membership in the A.A.M.H. All new members will spend one year in Associate Membership. There are two levels of membership.

Associate Membership is open to those professionals who meet the degree requirements and have an interest in hypnosis and hypnoanalysis and desire membership in the Academy.

Clinical Membership is open to those professionals who meet the degree requirements, and have completed the Clinical Training Program (or its equivalent) and denote 50 percent or more of their clinical practice to hypnoanalysis. Elevation to Clinical Membership can be applied for one year after having become an Associate Member by filling out the appropriate forms.

Membership Entitles You To:

- Subscription to the *Medical Hypnoanalysis Journal.*
- Reduced registration fees at all A.A.M.H. seminars.
- Periodic informative newsletter containing announcements of upcoming events and shared insights.
- National Professional Referral/Service with a toll free 800 line.
- Membership directory.
- An opportunity to contribute to A.A.M.H. by participating actively in the organization, as a Board Member, Committee Member, or Task Force Member.

A Clinical Training Program is available through the A.A.M.H. for qualified therapists to become Medical Hypnoanalysts. Further information on training can be obtained throughout the A.A.M.H.

For further information on membership, *Medical Hypnoanalysis Journal,* or the A.A.M.H. Clinical Training Program call 1-800-34-H.Y.P.N.O. or write the A.A.M.H., 710 E. Ogden Avenue, Ste. 208, Naperville, IL 60563.

Special Offers:

20% Discount

On any products offered by Ryan Elliott, M.S.W., Thunderbird Circle Publishing. This one time offer is good for cassette tapes, books, and videos to the buyer of *Wide Awake, Clear Headed, and Refreshed . . .* only.

$85 VALUE **$85 VALUE**

Free Consultation

To original buyer of *Wide Awake, Clear Headed, and Refreshed . . .*, simply write me a 1 page letter describing your problem, phobia, dilemma or whatever you would like help with and I will write back within 4-6 weeks.

Send your letter to: Ryan Elliott, P.O. Box 535, Winfield, IL 60190.

Please do not call; limit your letter to 1 page.

Include this Coupon

❑ **Put me on your mailing list!**

Name ______________________________

Address ______________________________

City ____________________ Zip ____________

Phone (______) ______________________________

END NOTES

Chapter One

1. Case studies drawn from my files will be included throughout this work. In each instance, fictitious names or initials have been used to protect client identity.
2. *The Thompson Chain-Reference Bible, New International Version*, Matt. 22:36–40 (Grand Rapids, Michigan: B.B. Kirkbride Bible Co., Inc., 1987).

Chapter Two

1. Dracula movies portray hypnosis as Count Dracula's tool for controlling people. If you know a movie producer, please give him or her this book so he or she can get the facts straight. Let me know and I'll send you another copy free.
2. Joseph Murphy, D.R.S., Ph.D., D.D., L.L.D., *The Power of Your Subconscious Mind* (Englewood Cliffs, N.J.: Prentice-Hall, Inc., 1987), p. 35.
3. *Encyclopedia Britannica* (1979), vol. 9, pp. 133–140.
4. William J. Bryan, Jr., M.D., in letter to Dr. Chong Tong Mun of Singapore, Malaya, *The Journal of the American Institute of Hypnosis* (Jan. 1963): p. 4.
5. Dr. Bruce Goldberg, *Past Lives Future Lives* (North Hollywood, California: Newcastle Publishing Co., Inc., 1982), p. 14.
6. Ibid., p. 22.
7. Arthur S. Freeze, "The Power of Hypnosis," *Arthritis Today* (Jan.-Feb., 1988): p. 10.

8. Herbert Benson, M.D., *The Relaxation Response* (New York: Avon Books, by arrangement with William Morrow and Company Inc., New York, 1975), p. 101.
9. Ibid., p. 24.
10. Ibid., p. 25.
11. Ibid.

Chapter Three

1. David Boxerman and Aron Spilken, *Alpha Brain Waves*, (Milbrae, California: Celestial Arts, 1975), p. 12.
2. Ibid.
3. The word-association test works on the mathematical principle that if A=B and B=C, then A=C.
4. In my practice, I deal with different religious denominations and help the spiritually depressed reunite with their conceptions of the higher power.
5. Reported by Ellen J. Langer, Ph.D., in *Mindfulness* (Reading, Massachusetts: Addison-Wesley Publishing Co., 1989), and excerpted in *Psychology Today* (April 1989): p. 51.
6. Barbara Reynolds, "Treat Whole Person, Not Just the Disease," *USA Today*, Jan. 4, 1990, sec. A, p. 11.
7. Ibid.
8. Ibid.
9. Robert Ornstein, Ph.D., and David Sobel, M.D., *The Healing Brain* (New York: Simon & Schuster Inc., 1987), pp. 88–97.

Chapter Four

1. *Webster's New Collegiate Dictionary* (Springfield, Massachusetts: G.& C. Merriam Company, 1981), p. 509.
2. An antigen, in medicine, is a toxin or enzyme capable of stimulating an immune response.
3. From a tape of a Bryan course in hypnoanalysis given in 1973, "The Bryan Method of Hypnoanalysis" (Clinton, Missouri: Christopher M. D'Aunoy, 1979).
4. Ibid.
5. Ibid.

6. Ibid.
7. Ibid.

Chapter Five

1. Hans Selye, M.D., *The Stress of Life*, rev. ed. (New York: McGraw-Hill Book Co., 1978), p. 1.
2. Peter Brill, M.D., and John P. Hayes, *Taming Your Turmoil* (Englewood Cliffs, N. J.: Prentice Hall, Inc., 1981), pp. 128–29.
3. Greg Risberg presented a seminar on touching at the Single Professional's Society at the Glen Ellyn Holiday Inn in 1987.
4. Louis K. Boswell, M.D., "Baby Stress," *Subconsciously Speaking* (Spring/Summer 1988): p. 1.
5. Ibid., p. 7.

Chapter Six

1. Serge King, *Imagineering for Health* (Wheaton, Illinois: The Theosophical Publishing House, 1980), pp. 16–18.
2. Charles M. Citrenbaum, Mark E. King, and William I. Cohen, *Modern Clinical Hypnosis for Habit Control* (New York: W. W. Norton & Company, 1985), p. 35.
3. Erich Fromm wrote a book about this called *Escape from Freedom* (New York: Avon Books, 1982).
4. Thomas Budzynski, "Tuning in on the Twilight Zone," *Psychology Today* 11, no. 3 (Aug. 1977): pp. 40–41.
5. Ibid., p. 40.
6. Ibid.
7. Ibid., p. 41.
8. Dr. Leo Louis Martello, "Sleep Learning: Education of the Future," *The New Journal of Hypnotism* (June 1988): pp. 16–18.
9. Ibid., p. 16.
10. This exercise came to me from Jackie Tschetter, a workshop leader and lay hypnotist.
11. Charles Thomas Cayce suggested this in a seminar I attended at the Unity of Oak Park in 1989.

Chapter Seven

1. Philip M. Bonelli, M.A., "Smoking Therapy: A Composite Approach," *Journal of Medical Hypnoanalysis* (Nov. 1980): p. 165.
2. From Ellen J. Langer, Ph.D., *Mindfulness*. (Reading, Massachusetts: Addision-Wesley Publishing Co., 1989), as quoted in *Psychology Today* (April 1989): p. 51.
3. *Small Business Report*, July 1985, p. 91.

Chapter Eight

1. The first three letters of diet spell "die," and who wants to die; consequently, the idea of dieting triggers a survival response.
2. Louis K. Boswell, "Eating Poor, Feeling Poor," *Subconsciously Speaking* (Winter 1987): p. 4.
3. Ryan Elliott, "Past Life Regression in Treating a Ponce de Leon Syndrome," *Medical Hypnoanalysis Journal* 2, no. 4, (Dec. 1987): pp. 148–50.
4. William J. Bryan, Jr., M.D., "Ponce de Leon Syndrome," *Journal of the American Institute of Hypnosis* 5, no. 1 (Jan. 1965): pp. 34-43.
5. William J. Bryan, Jr., M.D., "The Walking Zombie Syndrome." *Journal of the American Institute of Hypnosis* 2, no. 3 (Mar. 1961): pp. 10-18.

Chapter Nine

1. Arthur B. Hardy, M.D., *Everything You've Ever Wanted to Know about Phobias . . . But Had No One to Ask* (Menlo Park, California: Terraps Programs, 1989), p. 46.
2. Manuel D. Zane and Harry Milt, *Your Phobia: Understanding Your Fears through Contextual Therapy* (Washington, D.C.: American Psychiatric Press, 1984), p. 16.
3. Ibid., p. 64.
4. Nicholas Cooper-Lewter, M.S.W., ACSW, "Initial Environmental Experience: A Powerful Tool for Psychotherapy and Hypnotherapy," *Medical Hypnoanalysis* (Nov. 1981): p. 158.

5. Louis K. Boswell, "The Initial Sensitizing Event of Emotional Disorders," *British Journal of Medical Hypnotism* (Spring 1961): p. 12. As quoted in *Medical Hypnoanalysis* (Nov. 1981): p. 158.
6. Burton J. Rubin, *Stage Fright Handbook* (Saratoga Springs, New York: Decision-Making Systems, Ltd., 1986), p. 2.
7. Michael T. Motley, "Taking the Terror out of Talk," *Psychology Today* (Jan. 1988): p. 47.
8. Ibid., p. 48.
9. Ibid., p. 49.
10. Ibid.
11. Rubin, *Stage Fright Handbook*, pp. 28–47.
12. Denise Fortino, "Conquering Phobias," *New Woman*, May 1990, p. 125.
13. Rheta Grimsley Johnson, *Good Grief, The Story of Charles M. Schulz* (New York: Pharos Books, 1989), p. 38.
14. Ibid., p. 39.
15. Ann Landers, "Anxiety Attacks Need Right Professional Care," *Greensboro News and Record*, Jan. 25, 1990, sec. B, p. 3.
16. In many cases, by finding and understanding and undermining the negative suggestions, a single case of phobia or panic attack can be cleared up and resolved.

Chapter Ten

1. Melody Beattie, *Codependent No More* (New York: Harper & Row, by arrangement with the Hazelden Foundation, 1987), p. 33.
2. Donald Brennan, "The War for Codependents," *The Recovery Press*, April 1991, p. 16.
3. Angelyn Miller, *The Enabler: When Helping Harms the Ones You Love* (Austin, Texas: Hunter House, 1989), p. 7.
4. Ibid., p. 29.
5. Ibid.
6. Beattie, *Codependent No More*, p. 33.
7. Miller, *The Enabler*, p. 25.
8. Beattie, *Codependent No More*, pp. 37–45.

9. John Bradshaw, *Homecoming, Reclaiming and Championing Your Inner Child* (New York: Bantam Books, 1990), pp. 8–9.
10. John Scott, Sr., hypnosis script on identity problems.
11. Ibid.
12. John Bradshaw, *Religious Addiction*, a tape.
13. Ibid.
14. Ibid.
15. Ibid.
16. Joan Borysenko, Ph.D., “Getting Rid of Unhealthy Guilt,” *Shape*, Aug. 1990, p. 75.
17. Ibid.
18. Bradshaw, *Homecoming*, p. 21.
19. James F. Masterson, “The Hollow Self,” *Self*, Aug. 1990, p. 123.
20. From the pamphlet *Plain Talk About Depression*, published by the National Institute of Mental Health, Office of Scientific Information, 5600 Fishers Lane, Rockville, Maryland 20857.
21. From *Headlines*, published by Human Services, Inc., 4514 Travis, Suite 305, Dallas, Texas 75206. Copyright 1990. For more information call 1-800-873-2834.
22. Alcoholics Anonymous, P.O. Box 459, Grand Central Station, New York, New York 10163.
23. From the pamphlet *Letting Go of the Need to Control*, published in 1987 by the Hazelden Foundation, Center City, Minnesota 55012, p. 1.
24. Alcoholics Anonymous.
25. Miller, *The Enabler*, p. 91.
26. Gershen Kaufmann, *SHAME: The Power of Caring* (Cambridge, Massachusetts: Schenkman, 1990), p. 37.

Chapter Eleven

1. Joe Paterno with Bernard Asbell, *Paterno: By the Book* (New York: Random House, 1989), p. 81.
2. Roger Kahn, “They Ain’t Getting No Maiden,” in I Managed Good, But Boy Did They Play Bad, eds. Jim Bouton with Neil Offen (Chicago: Playboy Press, 1973), p. 172.

3. Les Cunningham and Wayne Ralph, *Hypnosport: How You Can Improve Your Sporting Performances* (Glendale, California: Westwood Publishing Company, 1981), p. 3.
4. Paterno with Asbell, *Paterno: By the Book*, pp. 129–30.
5. Ibid., p. 82.
6. Ibid., p. 94.
7. Ed Temple with B'Lou Carter, *Only the Pure in Heart Survive* (Nashville, Tennessee: Broadman Press, 1980), p. 54.
8. Willie Mays with Lou Sahadi, *Say Hey: The Autobiography of Willie Mays* (New York: Simon and Schuster, Inc., 1988), p. 15.
9. Ibid., pp. 72–73.
10. Cunningham and Ralph, *Hypnosport*, p. 140.
11. Ibid.
12. Ibid., pp. 140–141.
13. Ibid.
14. Ibid.
15. Ibid.
16. These principles are adapted from a script by the AAMH.
17. Tim Gallwey, *The Inner Game of Tennis* (New York: Random House, 1974).
18. James R. Rippe, M.D., and William Southmayd, M.D. *The Sports Performance Factors* (New York: Putnam Publishing Group, 1986).
19. Dr. Taylor told me about this case and gave me permission to use it.
20. Ibid., p. 3.
21. Eric Berne, M.D., *What Do You Say after You Say Hello?* (New York: Bantam Books, 1975), p. 205.

Chapter Twelve

1. Gerald May, *Care of Mind—Care of Spirit: Psychiatric Dimensions of Spiritual Direction* (New York: Harper and Row, 1982), p. 57.
2. Daniel A. Zelling, M.D., in an editorial in the *Journal of the American Academy of Medical Hypnoanalysts* 1, no. 2 (Dec. 1986): p. 46.

3. C. Alan Anderson, *The Problem Is God* (Walpole, New Hampshire: Stillpoint Publishing, 1984), p. 242.
4. Ibid., p. 241.
5. D. Scott Rogo, "Religion in America Today and the Vital Role of New Thought," *Science of Mind* (Oct. 1987): p. 10–12.
6. Ibid.
7. From 50 to 60 percent of my clients are Catholics, recovering Catholics, or retired Catholics.
8. Cassie recalled having her vaginal cavity probed by her mother's fingers.
9. *The Thompson Chain-Reference Bible, New International Version*, Gen. 1:27–28 (Grand Rapids, Michigan: B.B. Kirkbride Bible Co., Inc., 1987).
10. Ibid., Gal. 2:16.
11. Ibid., Gal. 2:21.
12. Ibid., Gal. 3:6.
13. Ibid., Gal. 3:16–18.
14. Ibid., Gal. 3:19.
15. Ibid., Gal. 3:24–26, 29.
16. I will not force a past-life regression or attempt to make a person believe in reincarnation. My job is not to proselytize but to analyze and remove negativity in pursuit of my client's goals.
17. Henry Reid, Ph.D., ed., "Confession Is Good for You," *Perspective on Consciousness and Psi Research* 7, no. 6 (April 1986): p. 3.
18. Thomas A. Ritzman, M.D., "Depression and the Nature of God," *Medical Hypnoanalysis* (Nov. 1982): p. 133.
19. *Thompson Bible*, Matt. 22:37–40.
20. In Anderson, *The Problem Is God,* n.p.
21. Ken Keyes, Jr., *The Hundredth Monkey* (Coos Bay, Oregon: Vision Books, Pocket Book ed., 1987). This is an interesting book, and I heartily recommend it.

INDEX

A

B

C

D

G

H

I

J

K

T

U

V

W

Z